SABISTON

REVIEW of SURGERY

SABISTON

REVIEW of SURGERY

Editor-in-Chief

Courtney M. Townsend, Jr., M.D.
Professor
John Woods Harris Distinguished Chairman
Department of Surgery
The University of Texas Medical Branch
Galveston, Texas

Associate Editors

R. Daniel Beauchamp, M.D.
The John L. Sawyers Professor of Surgery
Professor of Cell Biology
Chief, Division of Surgical Oncology
Department of Surgery
Associate Director of Clinical Programs
Vanderbilt Ingram Cancer Center
Vanderbilt University Medical Center
Vanderbilt University School of Medicine
Nashville, Tennessee

B. Mark Evers, M.D.
Professor and Robertson-Poth
Distinguished Chair in
General Surgery
Department of Surgery
The University of Texas Medical
Branch
Galveston, Texas

Kenneth L. Mattox, M.D.
Professor and Vice Chairman
Department of Surgery
Baylor College of Medicine
Chief of Staff
Chief of Surgery
Ben Taub General Hospital
Houston, Texas

W.B. SAUNDERS COMPANY
A Harcourt Health Sciences Company
Philadelphia London New York St. Louis Sydney Toronto

W.B. SAUNDERS COMPANY
A Harcourt Health Sciences Company

The Curtis Center
Independence Square West
Philadelphia, Pennsylvania 19106

Library of Congress Cataloging-in-Publication Data

Sabiston review of surgery. 3rd ed./editor-in-chief, Courtney M. Townsend, Jr.; associate editors, R. Daniel Beauchamp, B. Mark Evers, Kenneth L. Mattox.

p. cm.

Rev. ed. of: Review of surgery. 2nd ed. c1997.
To be used with: Textbook of surgery. 16th ed. c2001.

ISBN 0–7216–9258–3

1. Surgery—Examinations, questions, etc. 2. Surgery, Operative—Examinations, questions, etc. I. Title: Review of surgery. II. Townsend, Courtney M. III. Sabiston, David C. IV. Review of surgery. V. Textbook of surgery. [DNLM: 1. Surgery—Examination Questions. 2. Surgical Procedures, Operative—Examination Questions. WO 100 T3552 2001 Suppl.]

RD31.S23 2001 Suppl. 617′.0076–dc21

00–046406

Acquisitions Editor: Lisette Bralow
Developmental Editor: Janice Gaillard
Copy Editor: Mimi McGinnis
Production Manager: Frank Polizzano
Book Designer: Sasha O'Malley

SABISTON REVIEW OF SURGERY ISBN 0–7216–9258–3

Printed in the United States of America.

Last digit is the print number: 9 8 7 6 5 4 3 2 1

CONTRIBUTORS

STEVEN A. AHRENDT, M.D.
Medical College of Wisconsin

FRANK G. ALBERTA, M.D.
University of Connecticut Health Center

E. FRANÇOIS ALDRICH, M.D.
University of Maryland School of Medicine

SCOTT K. ALPARD, B.A.
The University of Texas Medical Branch

CARLOS ALVAREZ, M.D.
University of Medicine and Dentistry of New Jersey Medical School

DANA K. ANDERSEN, M.D.
Yale University School of Medicine

ROBERT W. ANDERSON, B.S. Eng., M.D., M.B.A.
Duke University School of Medicine

RICHARD J. ANDRASSY, M.D.
University of Texas–Houston Medical School

PETER B. ANGOOD, M.D.
Yale University School of Medicine

CLINTON K. ATKINSON, M.D.
East Carolina University School of Medicine

PAUL S. AUERBACH, M.D., M.S.
Stanford University School of Medicine

CLYDE F. BARKER, M.D.
University of Pennsylvania School of Medicine

BARBARA LEE BASS, M.D.
University of Maryland School of Medicine

R. DANIEL BEAUCHAMP, M.D.
Vanderbilt University School of Medicine

MICHAEL BELKIN, M.D.
Harvard Medical School

KENNETH L. BRAYMAN, M.D., PH.D.
University of Pennsylvania School of Medicine

MURRAY F. BRENNAN, M.D.
Weill Medical College of Cornell University

BRUCE D. BROWNER, M.D.
University of Connecticut Health Center

SUSAN I. BRUNDAGE, M.D., M.P.H.
Baylor College of Medicine

F. CHARLES BRUNICARDI, M.D.
Baylor College of Medicine

MARK P. CALLERY, M.D.
University of Massachusetts Medical School

JOHN L. CAMERON, M.D.
Johns Hopkins University School of Medicine

HERWIG CERWENKA, M.D.
Karl-Franzens University Medical School

RAVI S. CHARI, M.D.
University of Massachusetts Medical School

WILLIAM G. CHEADLE, M.D.
University of Louisville School of Medicine

EDWARD G. CHEKAN, M.D.
University of Virginia School of Medicine

LAURENCE Y. CHEUNG, M.D.
University of Kansas School of Medicine

LAWRENCE S. CHIN, M.D.
University of Maryland School of Medicine

WILLIAM G. CIOFFI, M.D.
Brown University School of Medicine

G. PATRICK CLAGETT, M.D.
University of Texas Southwestern Medical Center at Dallas

CHRISTINE S. COCANOUR, M.D.
University of Texas–Houston Medical School

RAUL COIMBRA, M.D.
University of California, San Diego, School of Medicine

ANTHONY J. COMEROTA, M.D.
Temple University School of Medicine

MICHAEL S. CONTE, M.D.
Harvard Medical School

MICHAEL S. COOKSON, M.D.
Vanderbilt University School of Medicine

CHARLES S. COX, JR., M.D.
University of Texas–Houston Medical School

CHAD E. DARLING, M.D.
University of Massachusetts Memorial Health Care

R. DUANE DAVIS, JR., M.D.
Duke University School of Medicine

ROMANO DELCORE, M.D.
University of Kansas School of Medicine

E. PATCHEN DELLINGER, M.D.
University of Washington School of Medicine

ARTHUR J. DIPATRI, M.D.
University of Maryland School of Medicine

GERARD M. DOHERTY, M.D.
Washington University School of Medicine

MICHELEA DOMENICK, M.D.
MCP–Hahnemann University Hospitals

MAGRUDER C. DONALDSON, M.D.
Harvard Medical School

ROGER R. DOZOIS, M.D., M.S.
Mayo Medical School

JONATHAN J. DRUMMOND-WEBB, M.B.B.CH.
Cleveland Clinic Foundation

DIANNE C. DUFFEY, M.D.
University of Texas Health Science Center at San Antonio

TIMOTHY J. EBERLEIN, M.D.
Washington University School of Medicine

HOWARD M. EISENBERG, M.D.
University of Maryland School of Medicine

SCOTT A. ENGUM, M.D.
Indiana University School of Medicine

ELOF ERIKSSON, M.D., PH.D.
Harvard Medical School

THOMAS R. EUBANKS, D.O.
University of Washington School of Medicine

W. STEVE EUBANKS, M.D.
Duke University School of Medicine

B. MARK EVERS, M.D.
The University of Texas Medical Branch

TIMOTHY C. FABIAN, M.D.
University of Tennessee Health Science Center

SAMIR M. FAKHRY, M.D.
Georgetown University School of Medicine and Health Sciences

MITCHELL P. FINK, M.D.
University of Pittsburgh School of Medicine

JOSEF E. FISCHER, M.D.
University of Cincinnati College of Medicine

GLEN A. FRANKLIN, M.D.
University of Louisville School of Medicine

DONALD E. FRY, M.D.
University of New Mexico School of Medicine

DAVID A. FULLERTON, M.D.
Northwestern University Medical School

PATRICIA C. FUREY, M.D.
Harvard Medical School

W. BARRITT GILBERT, M.D.
Vanderbilt University Medical Center

CYNTHIA A. GINGALEWSKI, M.D.
University of Connecticut School of Medicine

PETER S. GOEDEGEBUURE, PH.D.
Washington University School of Medicine

TOBY A. GORDON, SC.D.
Johns Hopkins University School of Medicine

DOUGLAS GOUMAS, M.D.
Orthopaedic Center, Nashua, New Hampshire

DARLA K. GRANGER, M.D.
University of Louisville School of Medicine

SEAN C. GRONDIN, M.D., M.P.H.
Harvard Medical School

JAY L. GROSFELD, M.D.
Indiana University School of Medicine

CARL E. HAISCH, M.D.
East Carolina University School of Medicine

CHARLES B. HAMMOND, M.D.
Duke University School of Medicine

JOHN B. HANKS, M.D.
University of Virginia School of Medicine

ALDEN H. HARKEN, M.D.
University of Colorado Health Sciences Center

DAVID T. HARRINGTON, M.D.
Brown University School of Medicine

JOHN H. HEALEY, M.D.
Weill Medical College of Cornell University

JOHN HENDRIX, M.D.
University of Virginia School of Medicine

DAVID N. HERNDON, M.D.
The University of Texas Medical Branch

BRADLEY B. HILL, M.D.
Stanford University School of Medicine

ASHER HIRSHBERG, M.D.
Baylor College of Medicine

MICHAEL D. HOLZMAN, M.D., M.P.H.
Vanderbilt University School of Medicine

DAVID B. HOYT, M.D.
University of California, San Diego, School of Medicine

J. DIRK IGLEHART, M.D.
Harvard Medical School

SUZANNE T. ILDSTAD, M.D.
University of Louisville School of Medicine

SANDEEP S. JEJURIKAR, M.D.
Good Samaritan Hospital, Downers Grove, Illinois

C. STARCK JOHNSON, M.D.
Brigham and Women's Hospital

R. SCOTT JONES, M.D.
University of Virginia School of Medicine

CAROLYN M. KAELIN, M.D.
Harvard Medical School

STEVEN A. KAGAN, M.D.
Temple University School of Medicine

ROBIN D. KIM, M.D.
University of Massachusetts Memorial Health Care

HAROLD E. KLEINERT, M.D.
University of Louisville School of Medicine

TIEN C. KO, M.D.
The University of Texas Medical Branch

TERRY C. LAIRMORE, M.D.
Washington University School of Medicine

KEVIN P. LALLY, M.D.
University of Texas–Houston Medical School

CHRISTINE L. LAU, M.D.
Duke University Medical Center

JONATHAN J. LEWIS, M.D., PH.D.
Weill Medical College of Cornell University

PAMELA A. LIPSETT, M.D.
Johns Hopkins University School of Medicine

JEANNE M. LUKANICH, M.D.
Harvard Medical School

JOHN S. MANCOLL, M.D.
Plastic Surgery Associates, Ft. Wayne, Indiana

JAMES F. MARKMANN, M.D., PH.D.
University of Pennsylvania School of Medicine

ROBERT G. MARVIN, M.D.
University of Texas–Houston Medical School

BRENT D. MATTHEWS, M.D.
Carolinas Medical Center

KENNETH L. MATTOX, M.D.
Baylor College of Medicine

RICHARD L. McCANN, M.D.
Duke University School of Medicine

JOHN C. McDONALD, M.D.
Louisiana State University Health Sciences Center

ROGER B. B. MEE, CH.B., M.B.
Cleveland Clinic Foundation

WILLIAM C. MEYERS, M.D.
University of Massachusetts Medical School

CARMELO A. MILANO, M.D.
Duke University School of Medicine

CHARLES C. MILLER III, PH.D.
University of Texas Health Sciences Center at Houston Medical School

JOHN H. MILLER, M.D.
The University of Texas Medical Branch

JEFFREY F. MOLEY, M.D.
Washington University School of Medicine

FREDERICK A. MOORE, M.D.
University of Texas–Houston Medical School

RICHARD J. MULLINS, M.D.
Oregon Health Sciences University School of Medicine

ALI NAJI, M.D., PH.D.
University of Pennsylvania School of Medicine

ELAINE E. NELSON, M.D.
San Jose Medical Center

HEIDI NELSON, M.D.
Mayo Medical School

ROBERT L. NORRIS, M.D.
Stanford University School of Medicine

KIM M. OLTHOFF, M.D.
University of Pennsylvania School of Medicine

MARK B. ORRINGER, M.D.
University of Michigan School of Medicine

THEODORE N. PAPPAS, M.D., M.S.
Duke University School of Medicine

CARLOS A. PELLEGRINI, M.D.
University of Washington School of Medicine

LINDA G. PHILLIPS, M.D.
The University of Texas Medical Branch

HENRY A. PITT, M.D.
Medical College of Wisconsin

HIRAM C. POLK, JR., M.D.
University of Louisville School of Medicine

HANS STEFAN PREUSS, M.D.
Harvard Medical School

DONALD S. PROUGH, M.D.
The University of Texas Medical Branch

JOE B. PUTNAM, JR., M.D.
The University of Texas M. D. Anderson Cancer Center

PATRICK R. REARDON, M.D.
Baylor College of Medicine

ROCCO RICCIARDI, M.D.
University of Massachusetts Memorial Health Care

LAYTON F. RIKKERS, M.D.
University of Wisconsin School of Medicine

MICHAEL S. ROHR, M.D., PH.D.
Bowman Gray School of Medicine

ROLANDO H. ROLANDELLI, M.D.
Temple University School of Medicine

RONNIE A. ROSENTHAL, M.D.
Yale University School of Medicine

EDMUND J. RUTHERFORD, M.D.
University of North Carolina at Chapel Hill School of Medicine

HAZIM J. SAFI, M.D.
University of Texas Health Sciences Center at Houston Medical School

BRADLEY K. SCHAFFER, M.D.
University of Massachusetts Memorial Health Care

BRUCE DAVID SCHIRMER, M.D.
University of Virginia School of Medicine

HILLIARD F. SEIGLER, M.D.
Duke University School of Medicine

SHIMUL A. SHAH, M.D.
University of Massachusetts Memorial Health Care

ABRAHAM SHAKED, M.D., PH.D.
University of Pennsylvania School of Medicine

GEORGE F. SHELDON, M.D.
University of North Carolina at Chapel Hill School of Medicine

EDWARD R. SHERWOOD, M.D., PH.D.
The University of Texas Medical Branch

KEVIN M. SITTIG, M.D.
Louisiana State University Health Sciences Center

CRAIG L. SLINGLUFF, JR., M.D.
University of Virginia School of Medicine

JOSEPH A. SMITH, JR., M.D.
Vanderbilt University School of Medicine

JULIE ANN SOSA, M.D.
Johns Hopkins University School of Medicine

JAMES D. ST. LOUIS, M.D.
Duke University Medical Center

DAVID J. SUGARBAKER, M.D.
Harvard Medical School

JAMES C. THOMPSON, M.D.
The University of Texas Medical Branch

COURTNEY M. TOWNSEND, JR., M.D.
The University of Texas Medical Branch

GILBERT R. UPCHURCH, Jr., M.D.
University of Michigan Medical School

RANDAL S. WEBER, M.D.
University of Pennsylvania School of Medicine

SAMUEL A. WELLS, Jr., M.D.
Washington University School of Medicine

ANTHONY D. WHITTEMORE, M.D.
Harvard Medical School

BRADON J. WILHELMI, M.D.
Southern Illinois University School of Medicine

ROBERT J. WINCHELL, M.D.
University of California, San Diego, School of Medicine

STEVEN E. WOLF, M.D.
The University of Texas Medical Branch

YEHUDA G. WOLF, M.D.
Hadassah Medical School

PO-SHENG YANG, M.D.
Sun Yat-Sen Cancer Center, Koo Foundation

CHARLES J. YEO, M.D.
Johns Hopkins University School of Medicine

CHRISTOPHER K. ZARINS, M.D.
Stanford University School of Medicine

MICHAEL E. ZENILMAN, M.D.
Albert Einstein College of Medicine of Yeshiva University

JOSEPH B. ZWISCHENBERGER, M.D.
The University of Texas Medical Branch

PREFACE

The *Review of Surgery* is designed to provide medical students, residents, and practicing surgeons the best tool for preparation for any challenge in surgery. One will be able to assess and expand one's knowledge from more than 1200 review questions prepared by national and international authorities who are thoroughly familiar with their fields. Answers and complete rationales have been provided. The questions and analyses present specific numbers in the *Sabiston Textbook of Surgery,* 16th edition, so that self-directed, in-depth study of particular areas can more easily and efficiently be carried out.

Medical students preparing for rounds and oral and written examinations, house officers preparing for in-training and certifying examinations, and practicing physicians preparing for recertification examinations will find this *Review* most helpful for their efforts. In this edition, questions involving various surgical specialties, including neurosurgery, orthopaedics, otolaryngology, pediatric surgery, plastic, maxillofacial, and hand surgery, gynecology, and urology, are discussed in detail; the *Review of Surgery* will be useful for preparation for these specialty board examinations as well as for vascular surgery, pediatric surgery, and colon and rectal surgery. The *Review of Surgery* is a comprehensive, relevant teaching device that reflects all of the updates, developments, and new information that make the *Sabiston Textbook of Surgery,* 16th edition, a definitive reference in the field.

Courtney M. Townsend, Jr., M.D.

NOTICE

Medicine is an ever-changing field. Standard safety precautions must be followed, but as new research and clinical experience broaden our knowledge, changes in treatment and drug therapy may become necessary or appropriate. Readers are advised to check the most current product information provided by the manufacturer of each drug to be administered to verify the recommended dose, the method and duration of administration, and contraindications. It is the responsibility of the treating physician, relying on experience and knowledge of the patient, to determine dosages and the best treatment for each individual patient. Neither the Publisher nor the editor assumes any liability for any injury and/or damage to persons or property arising from this publication.

THE PUBLISHER

CONTENTS

CHAPTER 1

BASIC SCIENCE IN SURGERY

1. The human genome is encoded in:

A. Proteins.
B. DNA.
C. RNA.
D. Histones.

DISCUSSION: The entire human genetic information, or human genome, is encoded in the nucleotide bases of deoxyribonucleic acid (DNA). This genetic information is translated into ribonucleic acid (RNA) and then protein, leading to the expression of specific biological characteristics or phenotypes.
Textbook: Pages 13–14 ANSWER: B

2. What is the most important step in the control of gene expression?

A. RNA stability.
B. Protein translation.
C. RNA processing.
D. Gene transcription.

DISCUSSION: Gene expression can be controlled at six major steps in the synthetic pathway from DNA to RNA to protein. The first and most important control of gene expression is at the level of gene transcription, which determines when and how often a given gene is transcribed into RNA molecules.
Textbook: Page 16 ANSWER: D

3. The most important recombinant DNA technology includes all of the following except:

A. Microinjection of genetic information.
B. Determination of the nucleotide sequences.
C. Rapid amplification of DNA sequences.
D. Cutting DNA at specific sites by restriction nucleases.

DISCUSSION: The most important recombinant DNA technology includes the ability to cut DNA at specific sites by restriction nucleases, to rapidly amplify DNA sequences, to rapidly determine the nucleotide sequences, to clone a DNA fragment, and to create a DNA sequence.
Textbook: Page 17 ANSWER: A

4. Which family of proteins is involved in the execution of apoptosis?

A. Cyclin-dependent kinases.
B. G proteins.
C. Caspases.
D. Histones.

DISCUSSION: Caspases, or *c*ysteine *asp*artate prote*ases*, are a highly conserved family of proteins that is involved in the execution of apoptosis. These enzymes cleave specific protein substrates leading to the morphologic and biochemical features seen in apoptotic cells.
Textbook: Page 21 ANSWER: C

5. The predominant action of interleukin-10 (IL-10) is to:

A. Increase production of pro-inflammatory cytokines by monocytes and macrophages.
B. Induce fever.
C. Induce apoptosis.
D. Decrease production of pro-inflammatory cytokines by monocytes and macrophages.
E. Induce angiogenesis in healing wounds.

DISCUSSION: IL-4, IL-13, and especially IL-10 are predominantly anti-inflammatory cytokines. All three of these cytokines are produced by T-helper 2 (Th2) cells, and among other roles, serve to modulate the production of pro-inflammatory cytokines, like tumor necrosis factor and IL-1, by macrophages and monocytes.
Textbook: Page 38 ANSWER: D

6. When human subjects are injected with recombinant IL-1β, which of the following effects is observed?

A. Thrombocytopenia.
B. Hypertension.
C. Increased appetite.
D. Hyperferremia.
E. Fever.

DISCUSSION: IL-1β is a potent pyrogen. Some other effects of IL-1β include the induction of hypoferremia, suppression of appetite, systemic arterial hypotension, and induction of thrombocytosis.
Textbook: Page 33 ANSWER: E

7. Which of the following agents has been shown to improve survival in humans with sepsis or septic shock?

A. Recombinant human interleukin-1 receptor antagonist.

B. Monoclonal anti–tumor necrosis factor (TNF) antibodies.
C. Glucocorticoids.
D. Soluble TNF receptor fusion proteins.
E. None of the above.

DISCUSSION: To date, no form of "adjuvant therapy" has been shown to clearly improve survival in patients with sepsis or septic shock. Although in some cases post-hoc analyses have shown some evidence of benefit for certain subsets of patients, the results of trials with recombinant human interleukin-1 receptor antagonist, various monoclonal anti-TNF antibodies, high doses of glucocorticoids, and various soluble TNF receptor fusion proteins have all been negative when analyzed on an intent-to-treat basis.

Textbook: Page 35 ANSWER: E

8. The intracellular signal transduction pathway activated by binding of lipopolysaccharide (LPS) to its receptor (CD14) is very similar to the signal transduction pathway triggered by binding of which cytokine to its receptor?

A. Interleukin-1 (IL-1).
B. Interferon gamma.
C. Tumor necrosis factor.
D. IL-6.
E. IL-8.

DISCUSSION: Major elements of the IL-1 signal transduction pathway have been shown to be important in the mechanism whereby inflammatory cells respond to LPS (endotoxin from gram-negative bacteria). The signaling components of the LPS receptor are orthologs of a protein called Toll originally described in the fruit fly, *Drosophila melanogaster.* At least one of these proteins, Tlr4, uses key components of the signal transduction apparatus employed by the IL-1 receptor, including MyD88 and interleukin receptor-associated kinase (IRAK), to initiate intracellular responses to LPS.

Textbook: Page 33 ANSWER: A

9. Circulating levels of which cytokine are commonly elevated in patients with sepsis?

A. Interleukin-1 (IL-1).
B. IL-6.
C. IL-12.
D. IL-18.
E. Interferon-gamma (IFN-γ).

DISCUSSION: Circulating concentrations of IL-6 are markedly elevated in patients with sepsis. Moreover, plasma levels of this cytokine tend to correlate directly with the risk of death in patients with sepsis or septic shock. Although detectable concentrations of IL-1, IL-12, or IFN-γ are occasionally reported in critically ill patients, for the most part, circulating levels of these cytokines are too low to be detectable even in patients with overwhelming infections.

Textbook: Page 37 ANSWER: B

NOTES

NOTES

CHAPTER 2

SURGICAL PRINCIPLES

1. The biochemical factor that most rapidly influences the distribution of water between the intracellular and extracellular compartments is which of the following?

A. Permeability of the cell membrane to sodium.
B. Plasma oncotic pressure.
C. Osmotic forces that achieve an equilibrium of intracellular and extracellular fluid osmolality.
D. Urea concentration in the extracellular fluid.

DISCUSSION: Water meets negligible resistance crossing cell membranes, and when there is a change in the osmolality in either the extracellular or intracellular compartment, water quickly is shifted by osmotic forces to achieve a new equilibrium. Although sodium is the dominant extracellular fluid osmole, the transport of sodium across the cell membrane is a complex active process that requires time and is slow compared with the rapid movement of water when osmolality changes. Oncotic pressure refers to the osmotic pressure caused by very large solutes such as proteins and is not a principal factor in determining water balance between the cell and extracellular fluid. Urea is not a major factor in moving water across the cell membrane because the cell membrane is as permeable to urea as to water.

Textbook: Page 46 ANSWER: C

2. Patients who have advanced cirrhosis of the liver and tense ascites and who then develop hyponatremia most commonly have as an origin for their electrolyte abnormality:

A. A contracted extracellular volume.
B. An expanded plasma volume.
C. A sudden decline in glomerular filtration rate.
D. A contracted vascular volume.

DISCUSSION: The pathophysiologic problem for patients with cirrhosis of the liver is that with portal hypertension sodium and water are retained as ascites, thus causing an expanded extracellular fluid volume. The plasma volume may or may not be expanded depending on the hematocrit, but these patients do typically have a contracted total vascular volume. Endocrine, baroreceptor, and renal responses to a reduced blood volume have an influence on renal function. The nephrons retain water and sodium, despite the expanded extracellular compartment, exacerbating the ascites. Renal failure, defined as a critical reduction in glomerular filtration rate, may occur during the final stages as water overload causes tense ascites.

Textbook: Page 48 ANSWER: D

3. Which of the following factors would strongly favor an increased release of arginine vasopressin from the posterior pituitary?

A. An increase in serum osmolality.
B. Narcotic administration to the point of sedation.
C. An intravenous infusion of 1L of 0.45 normal saline into a normal adult.
D. Elevated circulating aldosterone levels.

DISCUSSION: The synthesis of arginine vasopressin in the hypothalamus, and its release from the posterior pituitary, is controlled by a number of factors. In normal circumstances the amount of arginine vasopressin released increases as serum osmolality exceeds 290 mOsm/L. Pain can be a powerful stimulant for arginine vasopressin release, and thus less should be released if there is optimal pain control using narcotics to the point that the patient is sedated. Intravenous infusion of hypotonic fluid should result in a diuresis in part because arginine vasopressin is suppressed. Elevated aldosterone, although contributing to antidiuresis and elevated in hypovolemic patients as is arginine vasopressin, does not strongly favor increased arginine vasopressin.

Textbook: Pages 46–47 ANSWER: A

4. Which of the following agents would you expect to be the most effective therapy for a patient with metastatic renal cell carcinoma and a serum calcium of 16.5 mg/dl?

A. Mannitol.
B. Penicillin G.
C. Bisphosphonates.
D. Growth hormone.

DISCUSSION: A forced diuresis can be effective therapy for rapid correction of severe hypercalcemia, but the diuresis should be accomplished by intravenous infusion of isotonic saline and, if a diuretic is added, administration of furosemide or bumetanide. The bisphosphonate class of drugs suppresses release of calcium from bone by the action of osteoclasts. Neither penicillin G nor growth hormone has a clinically important calcium-lowering effect.

Textbook: Page 53 ANSWER: C

5. Which of the following molecules is a principal buffer of increased hydrogen anion concentration in the intracellular fluid?

A. Chloride.
B. Dibasic phosphate.
C. Albumin.
D. Carbonic acid.

DISCUSSION: Phosphate ion species are present in high concentrations in intracellular fluid, and when more hydrogen ions are released, as occurs with a shift of ATP to ADP, these protons are linked to dibasic phosphate–producing monobasic phosphate. This buffering of pH does not occur with chloride. Albumin and chloride are principally in the extracellular fluid. Carbonic acid is the intermediate molecule produced when bicarbonate ion buffers a proton, and as such, it is not a buffer.

Textbook: Pages 57–61 ANSWER: B

6. Which of the following adverse events can be a consequence of the fall below 7.20 of a patient's plasma pH?

A. Oliguria.
B. Pulmonary bronchospasm.
C. Pulmonary artery hypertension.
D. Hypothermia.

DISCUSSION: Acidemia is well tolerated in most patients, but when the plasma pH is less than 7.20, adverse events include impaired myocardial contractility and pulmonary artery hypertension. Pulmonary bronchospasm has not been linked directly to severe acidemia. Oliguria from acute renal failure and hypothermia are conditions associated with acidemia, but are not a consequence of the fall in pH.

Textbook: Page 60 ANSWER: C

7. The hyperdynamic circulation, in which the cardiac index can be two to three times normal in patients who are in septic shock, can usually be attributed to which of the following?

A. Increased myocardial contractility.
B. Adrenal insufficiency and depressed levels of circulating endogenous catecholamines.
C. A direct influence of endotoxin on vascular smooth muscle.
D. Stimulation of endogenous inflammatory mediators with vasodilators.

DISCUSSION: The vasodilation, and reduction in calculated systemic vascular resistance, that occurs in patients with sepsis is not mediated by the endotoxin, but rather is attributed to inflammatory cytokines, bradykinin, and increased synthesis of nitric oxide. Careful study of myocardial performance in patients with hyperdynamic septic shock has revealed impaired contractility. Adrenal medullary infarction with loss of release of epinephrine is a rare complication of serious infection.

Textbook: Pages 63–64 ANSWER: D

8. The cell or cell component central to wound healing is:

A. B cells.
B. T cells.
C. Leukocytes.
D. Macrophages.
E. Platelets.

DISCUSSION: Only macrophages directly affect fibroblasts, keratinocytes, and endothelial cells. Wound healing is not impaired in patients with decreased levels of any of the other cells. Macrophages are the one type of cell that, if present in diminished numbers, will retard the wound healing process.

Textbook: Pages 133–134 ANSWER: D

9. Thromboxane causes:

A. Fibroblast chemotaxis.
B. Vasoconstriction.
C. Collagen cross-linking.
D. Endothelial proliferation.
E. Bacterial lysis.

DISCUSSION: Thromboxane causes vasoconstriction. It is not chemotactic or mitogenic and has no impact on collagen formation. Thromboxane is not bactericidal.

Textbook: Page 132 ANSWER: B

10. Iron deficiency has an impact on wound healing by decreasing:

A. Early tensile strength.
B. DNA synthesis.
C. Conversion of hydroxyproline to proline.
D. Tissue oxygenation.
E. Fibroblast proliferation.

DISCUSSION: Iron deficiency has only a transient and reversible effect on wound healing strength, despite the dogma of the effect of anemia. It is not really known what the cause of the decreased early tensile strength is, but it does not appear to have an effect on DNA synthesis, tissue oxygenation, proliferation of any of the cells locally, or formation of collagen.

Textbook: Page 141 ANSWER: A

11. Hypertrophic scar is:

A. Another term for keloids.
B. More likely to occur on the face.
C. Genetic in origin.
D. Preventable.
E. Worsened with glucocorticoids.

DISCUSSION: Hypertrophic scar, unlike keloid scar, is preventable. Keloids are not microscopically identical to hypertrophic scar and are genetic in origin, while hypertrophic scar is not. Both types of proliferative scar can be improved with topical or injectable glucocorticoid use. Hypertrophic scar tends to occur in areas of tension with poor approximation of the dermis or in areas where infection has occurred.

Textbook: Pages 139–140 ANSWER: D

12. The effects of diabetes on wound healing include:

A. Slowed epithelialization.
B. Reduced phagocytosis.
C. Glycosylated collagen.
D. Thickened basement membrane.
E. All of the above.

DISCUSSION: The effects of diabetes include all of the above answers. Likely, this is due to the hyperglycemia, which causes stiffening of all proteins as the excess glucose bonds to the protein structure. Therefore, all phases of wound healing are impaired.

Textbook: Page 141 ANSWER: E

13. Ionizing radiation causes hypoxia by:

A. Direct cellular injury to endothelium.
B. Basal membrane injury.
C. Release of histamine and serotonin.
D. Preventing the hypoxic stimulus of angiogenesis.
E. Increased dermal fibrosis and thickening.

DISCUSSION: Ionizing radiation prevents the hypoxic stimulus of angiogenesis. Although dermal fibrosis and thickening occurs, this does not cause hypoxia. No sufficient number of endothelial cells is injured to affect hypoxia. The release of histamine and serotonin, if anything, would serve as causes of angiogenesis.

Textbook: Page 141 ANSWER: D

14. Nicotine ingestion affects wound healing by:

A. Increasing fibroblast proliferation.
B. Increasing platelet adhesion.
C. Competitively competing with oxygen.
D. Inhibiting oxidative metabolism.
E. Inhibiting oxygen transport.

DISCUSSION: The direct effect of nicotine ingestion is to increase platelet adhesion. Nicotine also causes direct vasoconstriction. Thus, the net effect is primarily clogging of the capillary bed due to platelet adhesion. There is no competitive binding with oxygen or inhibition of oxidative metabolism or transport to have a direct effect on wound healing.

Textbook: Page 141 ANSWER: B

15. Which of the following events occurs in the proliferative phase of wound healing?

A. Histamine release.
B. Collagen cross-linking.
C. Thromboxane release.
D. Phagocytosis.
E. Collagen synthesis.

DISCUSSION: The proliferative phase includes chemotaxis and mitogenesis of the fibroblasts, keratinocytes, and endothelial cells. In addition, there is synthesis of collagen, elastic fibers, and glycosaminoglycans. In the inflammatory phase, there is release of histamine, thromboxane, and other inflammatory mediators. Phagocytosis of bacteria and necrotic tissue is caused by leukocytes, lymphocytes, keratinocytes, and macrophages. Collagen cross-linking does not occur until the maturational phase.

Textbook: Pages 134, 136–137 ANSWER: E

16. Chronic wounds characteristically have:

A. Tissue inflammation.
B. Decreased tissue inhibitor metalloprotease levels.
C. Increased gelatinase levels.
D. Increased collagenase levels.
E. All of the above.

DISCUSSION: Chronic wounds are now known to have certain characteristics distinctly different from acute wounds. There is an increased level in the matrix metalloproteases gelatinase and collagenase. At the same time, there is a decrease in the amount of tissue inhibitors of metalloproteases (TIMP). Inflammation characterizes these chronically open wounds that have not proceeded to closure.

Textbook: Page 203 ANSWER: E

17. The wound healing impairment caused by corticosteroid administration can be reversed by:

A. Vitamin A.
B. Vitamin C.
C. Zinc.
D. Vitamin K.
E. Vitamin B_{12}.

DISCUSSION: Corticosteroids appear to impair wound healing by stabilizing the lysosomal membranes. Vitamin A destabilizes the same membranes and appears to have a reverse effect on wound healing as a result. Patients who are chronically administered systemic corticosteroids can be treated by the administration of 25,000 units of vitamin A daily given orally. Vitamin C and zinc are coenzymes for collagen synthesis. Vitamin K is a coagulation factor. Vitamin B_{12} is essential to prevent megaloblastic anemia.

Textbook: Page 141 ANSWER: A

18. Which of the following glycosaminoglycans is not a component of skin?

A. Hyaluronic acid.
B. Chondroitin sulfate.
C. Dermatan sulfate.
D. Heparin sulfate.
E. Heparin.

DISCUSSION: All of the above-listed glycosaminoglycans are components of skin with the exception of heparin sulfate. Keratan sulfate also is not present in skin.

Textbook: Pages 135–136 ANSWER: D

19. The vast majority of human collagen is:

A. Type I.

B. Type III.
C. Type IV.
D. Type V.
E. Type VII.

DISCUSSION: Ninety percent of all human collagen is Type I.

Textbook: Page 136 ANSWER: A

20. When the fibroblast is arrested in the G_0 phase of replication, it can be made competent by:

A. Insulin-like growth factor-1 (IGF-1).
B. IGF-2.
C. Transforming growth factor-β (TGF-β).
D. Platelet-derived growth factor (PDGF).
E. Epidermal growth factor (EGF).

DISCUSSION: The fibroblast is made competent for replication by PDGF as well as basic fibroblast growth factor. Once competent, the fibroblast is stimulated to replicate by IGF and EGF. TGF-β stimulates collagen synthesis.

Textbook: Page 135 ANSWER: D

21. Endothelial cells are induced to form tubules by:

A. Vascular endothelial growth factor (VEGF).
B. Hypoxia.
C. Tumor necrosis factor-alpha (TNF-alpha).
D. Transforming growth factor-α (TGF-α).
E. Basic fibroblast growth factor (bFGF).

DISCUSSION: Both the presence of collagen fibers and TNF-α stimulate capillary tubule formation by endothelial cells. TGF-α stimulates endothelial cell proliferation. It is bFGF that begins the angiogenic cascade. Hypoxia causes the fibroblast to form more VEGF, which is mitogenic and chemotactic to endothelial cells.

Textbook: Pages 134–135 ANSWER: C

22. The *P* value of a randomized controlled clinical trial comparing operation A (new procedure) and operation B is .04. From this we can conclude that:

A. The Type II error is small and we can accept the findings of the study.
B. The probability of a false-negative conclusion that operation A is better than operation B when in truth it is not is 4%.
C. The power of the study to detect a difference between operation A and operation B is 96%.
D. The probability of a false-positive conclusion that operation A is better than operation B when in truth it is not is 4%.

DISCUSSION: The *P* value, or alpha, is the probability that a false-positive conclusion is selected when in truth it is not is called a Type I error. The erroneous false-negative conclusion is called a Type II (or beta) error. The probability of drawing a true-positive conclusion when this is correct is called the power of the study. By convention most studies use a 5% risk of concluding that experimental therapy and conventional therapy produce different clinical outcomes when in fact they do not (a false-positive, Type I, or alpha error of .05) and run a 20% risk of concluding that experimental therapy and conventional therapy do not produce clinical outcomes when in fact they do (a false-negative, Type II, or beta error of .2). The power of the study is then 1 to 0.20 or 80% chance of finding a difference between two therapies and of finding a statistical difference.

Textbook: Pages 153–154 ANSWER: D

23. A randomized clinical trial studies functional outcome of patients after coronary artery bypass surgery. The scores obtained from patients vary from 0 to 100 with a wide variation in values that are not easily predicted based on clinical assessment. You would like to know if the outcome in Patient Group A is different from that in Patient Group B. A reasonable statistical test to measure the differences between Patient Group A and Patient Group B is:

A. The Mann-Whitney test, because it measures data from two groups that are not normally distributed.
B. The chi-square test, because two groups are being studied and the proportion of patients having one outcome versus another is examined.
C. The *t* test, because two groups are compared and numerical data are involved.
D. The Pearson correlation coefficient.
E. Analysis of variance (ANOVA).

DISCUSSION: The Mann-Whitney test is appropriate when data are not normally distributed, that is, a nonparametric test versus a *t* test, which would be applied for normally distributed data. A chi-square test looks at frequency values between the two groups. Analysis of variance examines the differences between more than two groups.

Textbook: Page 153 ANSWER: A

24. A case series of 400 consecutive surgical procedures done at a single institution reports no mortality and minimal morbidity over a 10-year period compared with previous patients at that institution and with the literature. In critically appraising the article you recognize that:

A. The results of the study are so compelling that you should immediately change your technique because the results are much better than the results you currently achieve.
B. Changes in surgical care have occurred over time and therefore the results are completely explainable by this difference and the study has no application to your practice.
C. Patients in this report appear similar to to the patients you see with this disease and therefore the results of the study should be applied to your patients.
D. Results of this study could be influenced by selection and information bias as well as the use of historical controls and therefore application of this information should be done recognizing these possibilities.

DISCUSSION: A case series even when large can introduce enormous bias into the literature and should be applied to practice with caution.
Textbook: Page 146 ANSWER: D

25. The efficacy of a new drug treatment A, which is given four times a day with food, is established in a large well-conceived population-based study. This means that:

A. Routine application of treatment A in your patients is likely to achieve the same results.
B. The effectiveness of treatment A in your practice may be different compared with the study, which was done under *ideal* circumstances.
C. The power of a population-based study means that the results are Level 1 evidence and should be similar to how the drug works in your patients.
D. Treatment A will likely work just as well when given three times a day with or without food.

DISCUSSION: Many clinical trials are efficacy studies that are conducted under ideal circumstances rather than under actual clinical practice. Differences in effectiveness and efficacy are seen with increasing complexity of treatment when compliance is an issue.
Textbook: Page 146 ANSWER: B

26. The degree to which a test measures what it is intended to measure is:

A. Responsiveness.
B. Reliability.
C. Sensitivity.
D. Specificity.
E. Validity.

DISCUSSION: Validity is the degree to which a test measures what it is intended to measure, whereas responsiveness is the ability of a test to detect clinically meaningful changes; it also measures a test's reliability, that is, the extent to which a test yields consistent results on repeated trials. Sensitivity is the ability of a test to find the disease in patients who have the disease, whereas specificity is the ability of a test to find who does not have the disease.
Textbook: Page 146 ANSWER: E

In the box below indicate the correct terms:
Choose from the terms below to find the correct term with the proper formula:

Disease Present	Disease Not Present	Total
A (True +)	B (False +)	
C (False −)	D (True −)	
A + C = All disease	B + D = No disease	All patients = A + B + C + D

27. ____ D/(B + D)
28. ____ D/(C + D)
29. ____ A/(A + C)
30. ____ A/(A + B)
31. ____ A + C/(A + B + C + D)

A. Specificity.
B. Sensitivity.
C. Prevalence.
D. Positive predictive value.
E. Negative predictive value.

Textbook: Pages 151–154 ANSWERS: 27. A; 28. E; 29. B; 30. D; 31. C

32. (True or False) Human immunodeficiency virus (HIV) is the greatest infectious risk of transfusion.

DISCUSSION: Although HIV is the infectious risk that is of greatest concern to the lay public, a patient is more likely to acquire and die from hepatitis than HIV.
Textbook: Pages 75–76 ANSWER: False

33. Complications of massive transfusion include all of the following except:

A. Acidosis.
B. Coagulopathy.
C. Hypothermia.
D. Hypercalcemia.
E. Alkalosis.

DISCUSSION: Acidosis is common initially following massive transfusion both because of the lactic acidosis that is usually present as well as the acidic medium of stored blood products. The citrate contained within blood products is then converted to sodium bicarbonate in the liver with a resultant alkalosis. The coagulopathy that occurs with massive transfusion is multifactorial and includes a dilutional thrombocytopenia and decreased factor levels. Perhaps the most important factor in the development of coagulopathy is the development of hypothermia. Significant degrees of hypothermia can occur with rapid transfusion of large volumes of cold blood products. This is exacerbated in patients with accelerated heat loss due to exposure and open body cavities. Citrate binds to calcium leading to transient hypocalcemia.
Textbook: Pages 74–75 ANSWER: D

34. Infectious risks of transfusion include all of the following except:

A. Hepatitis.
B. *Yersinia* infection.
C. Malaria.
D. Human immunodeficiency virus (HIV).
E. Cytomegalovirus (CMV).
F. None of the above.

DISCUSSION: HIV and hepatitis remain the most serious infectious risks of transfusion. Other infectious risks include CMV, Epstein-Barr virus, *Trypanosoma cruzi*, *Yersinia*, and malaria.
Textbook: Pages 75–76 ANSWER: F

35. The following are true regarding red blood cell transfusion except:

A. Blood should be transfused one unit at a time, followed by an assessment of benefit.

B. The patient should be involved in the transfusion decision.
C. Hemoglobin should be maintained higher than 10.0 g/dl.
D. Objective criteria of oxygen delivery include base deficit and lactic acidosis.
E. Blood transfusion is unwarranted to improve wound healing or the patient's sense of well-being.

DISCUSSION: The decision for transfusion should be based on the physiologic status of the patient rather than on a predetermined level of hemoglobin. These end-points include symptoms, vital signs, and end-organ perfusion, such as urine output, base deficit, and lactic acidosis. Because the risk is cumulative, a reassessment should be performed after each unit is transfused.
Textbook: Pages 70–72 ANSWER: C

36. Consequences of transfusion include all of the following except:

A. Improved transplant graft survival.
B. Increased infectious complications.
C. Immunosuppression.
D. Improved wound healing.
E. Worsened prognosis with colorectal carcinoma.

DISCUSSION: Transfusion depresses the immune response, resulting in improved transplant graft survival, increased infectious complications, and decreased time to recurrence for several oncologic conditions. Increased circulating red cell mass does not improve wound healing.
Textbook: Pages 75–76 ANSWER: D

37. Each of the following adversely affects (shift to the left) the oxygen-dissociation curve except:

A. Acidosis.
B. Hypothermia.
C. Decreased 2,3-diphosphoglycerate (2,3-DPG).
D. Decreased $PaCO_2$.
E. Increased pH.

DISCUSSION: Alkalosis, hypothermia, decreased 2,3-DPG, and decreased $PaCO_2$ all result in a leftward shift of the oxygen-dissociation curve resulting in increased binding of oxygen to hemoglobin. Acidosis causes a rightward shift and decreased binding of oxygen to hemoglobin.
Textbook: Pages 74–75, 394 ANSWER: A

38. A major problem in nutritional support is identifying patients at risk. Studies suggest that these patients can be identified. Which of the following findings identify the patient at risk?

A. Weight loss of greater than 10% over 2 to 4 months.
B. Serum albumin of less than 3 g per 100 ml in the hydrated state.
C. Malnutrition as identified by global assessment.
D. Serum transferrin of less than 220 mg per 100 ml.
E. All of the above.

DISCUSSION: All of these are at least partially correct. It is not clear whether weight loss of 10% or 15% is the required threshold, but it certainly is close. Serum albumin of less than 3 g per 100 ml remains the most constant identifier of patients at risk in the literature and has been so for years. Global assessment in the hands of an experienced investigator is quite efficacious at identifying persons at risk. Serum transferrin is certainly a confirmatory identifier of patients with malnutrition—and may be even a primary one.
Textbook: Pages 100–101 ANSWER: E

39. Essential fatty acid deficiency may complicate total parenteral nutrition (TPN). Which of the following statements is false?

A. Essential fatty acid deficiency may be prevented by the administration of 4 to 6% of total calories as fat emulsion.
B. Fat-free parenteral nutrition results in the appearance of plasma abnormalities, indicating essential fatty acid deficiency, within 7 to 10 days of initiation.
C. An abnormal plasma eicosatrienoic-arachidonic acid ratio is always associated with essential fatty acid deficiency.
D. Following initiation of fat-free parenteral nutrition, dry, scaly skin associated with a maculopapular rash indicates essential fatty acid deficiency.

DISCUSSION: Biochemical evidence of essential fatty acid deficiency may occur as early as 7 to 10 days following initiation of fat-free parenteral nutrition. The decrease in arachidonic acid in plasma and the appearance of the abnormal eicosatrienoic acid may yield the earliest indication of prostaglandin deficiency; it is not absolute. Decreased intraocular pressure, another early indication of prostaglandin deficiency, may appear as soon as 7 days following initiation of fat-free parenteral nutrition. Although my current practice is to give at least 500 ml of 10% lipid emulsion daily to provide 20 to 25% of total calories to support hepatic protein synthesis, as little as 4 to 6% of total daily calories as fat prevents essential fatty acid deficiency. Practically, this may be undertaken by the administration of 500 ml of 10% lipid three times weekly. The appearance of eicosatrienoic acid and a decrease in arachidonic acid, and a change in ratio, are not essential to the diagnosis of essential fatty acid deficiency, but this plasma abnormality is often present.
Textbook: Page 120 ANSWER: C

40. It is stated that enteral nutrition is safer than parenteral nutrition. Which of the following may be complications of enteral nutrition?

A. Hyperosmolar, nonketotic coma.
B. Vomiting and aspiration.

C. Pneumatosis cystoides intestinalis.
D. Perforation and peritonitis.
E. All of the above.

DISCUSSION: It is not necessarily true that enteral nutrition is safer than parenteral nutrition, and it may in fact be associated with a higher risk of death than parenteral nutrition. Specifically, a well-run parenteral nutrition service should not be associated with significant mortality, except for the occasional death due to undetected yeast infection. On the other hand, enteral nutrition, especially if not carried out safely, can result in significant mortality. The most common of the severe complications of enteral nutrition result from the gastrostomy, or tube feedings into the stomach. Sudden changes in gastric motility, such as those associated with sepsis, may result in aspiration. Nasoenteric or nasoduodenal tubes help prevent this complication, as does shutting off enteral feedings between the hours of 11 PM and 7 AM. It is also essential to keep the patient's head elevated 30 degrees. Also necessary is the use of extreme care when initiating enteral nutrition. If hypertonic material is given into the stomach, one can increase osmolality followed by an increase in volume. If, however, the material is given into the small bowel, volume must be increased first and then tonicity, with the expectation that osmolality greater than 400 or 500 mOsm per liter may never be achieved without provoking severe diarrhea. If care is not taken with the initiation of enteral nutrition, massive diarrhea may result, including fluid loss, the absorption of enormous amounts of carbohydrate into the circulation with inadequate fluid to support it, and the development of hyperosmolar, nonketotic coma. Alternatively, severe unremitting diarrhea may result in necrosis of the intestinal wall, the appearance of pneumatosis cystoides intestinalis, and, finally, perforation and death. All of these complications may be prevented by judicious use of enteral nutrition with the same care one uses for parenteral nutrition.

Textbook: Page 104 ANSWER: E

41. Essential amino acids have been advocated as standard therapy for renal failure. Which of the following statements is true?

A. Increased survival from acute renal failure has been reported with both essential and nonessential amino acid therapy of patients in renal failure.
B. Essential amino acids accelerate the rise of blood urea nitrogen (BUN) secondary to the appearance of decreased urea.
C. Essential amino acids and hypertonic dextrose are a convenient form of therapy for hyperkalemia.
D. Essential amino acids decrease BUN and creatinine to the same degree as solutions containing excessive nonessential amino acids.

DISCUSSION: Essential amino acids and hypertonic dextrose, as opposed to hypertonic dextrose alone, were reported (Abel and coworkers) to be associated with a decreased mortality rate in mostly surgical patients with acute tubular necrosis. The most significant improvement in mortality, as compared with the control group receiving only hypertonic dextrose, was among patients who required dialysis (i.e., the more severely affected patients). Another group responding favorably to treatment includes patients with nonoliguric renal failure whose need for dialysis is not clearly established. The effect of essential amino acids in preventing a rise in BUN, as well as its beneficial effect in preventing hyperkalemia, may obviate dialysis in such patients. With increasing amounts of nonessential amino acids, BUN increases, and thus, dialysis is required. Prospective randomized studies comparing the use of essential versus nonessential amino acids in patients with acute renal failure have not been carried out in sufficient numbers to yield answers to this question.

Textbook: Page 115 ANSWER: C

42. A modified amino acid solution with increased equimolar branched-chain amino acids and decreased aromatic amino acids has been proposed for patients with hepatic insufficiency. Which of the following statements is true?

A. This formulation is proposed for use in patients with fulminant hepatitis.
B. Nitrogen balance is achieved in such patients with amounts of 40 g of amino acids per 24 hours.
C. The use of 80 to 100 g of such solutions is associated with hepatic encephalopathy.
D. In some studies of surgical patients, improvements in mortality have been reported.

DISCUSSION: The use of modified amino acid solutions is based on the false neurotransmitter hypothesis of the cause of hepatic coma. According to this hypothesis, the imbalance between aromatic and branched-chain amino acids in the plasma results in abnormally high levels of the toxic aromatic amino acids in the brain, thus provoking hepatic encephalopathy. The use of modified amino acid mixtures, with glucose as the calorie base, has been associated in a number of studies with improvement in encephalopathy. Meta-analysis has concluded that the use of such solutions is indicated as therapy for hepatic encephalopathy but has been proposed only for hepatic encephalopathy complicating acute exacerbation of chronic liver disease. Although there are a few anecdotal reports of beneficial effects on hepatic encephalopathy of acute fulminant hepatitis, the use of such a solution has not been advocated, but such a modified solution is tolerated better than standard amino acid mixtures in patients requiring total parenteral nutrition. In some studies, particularly in complicated surgical cases, the use of a high-branched-chain, low-aromatic amino acid solution has been associated with lower mortality. These statements are true only for studies in which the modified solutions are given with hypertonic glucose as a calorie base. Studies in which lipid was the principal calorie source have not revealed such improvements in mortality. In some studies, giving an aromatic amino acid–deficient, branched-chain amino acid–enriched solution to patients about to undergo resection of the liver has proved particularly efficacious in a group of patients with cirrhosis, decreasing morbidity and showing a trend toward decreased mortality.

Textbook: Page 116 ANSWER: D

43. In the nutritional support of patients with cancer, which of the following statements is true?

A. Nutritional support benefits the patient's lean body mass but does not enable the tumor to grow.
B. In experimental animals, the growth of implanted tumors is directly proportional to the amount of calories and protein supplied.
C. Prospective randomized trials of nutritional support utilizing chemotherapy and radiation therapy have revealed benefits to patients receiving total parenteral nutrition (TPN).
D. Studies of nutritional support for patients with cancer about to undergo surgery revealed decreased morbidity and mortality, especially morbidity from sepsis.

DISCUSSION: The problem with the patient with cancer is a very vexing one. Clearly, one of the metabolic effects of cancer, cachexia, affects patients in the last quartile of their disease and makes such patients intolerant of chemotherapy, radiation therapy, and, in many cases, operative procedures. TPN has been proposed as a means of reversing cachexia and enabling patients to better tolerate surgery, chemotherapy, and radiation therapy. In experimental animals, it is clear that the provision of calories and protein, especially in excessive amounts, is associated with the more rapid growth of tumors and decreased survival, especially in the group that is overfed in the extreme. There is also evidence suggesting that overfeeding, or at least TPN, may result in increased tumor growth (or at least change cell kinetics) in patients who are overnourished with TPN. Of the randomized prospective trials that have been carried out, no trial using chemotherapy or radiation therapy has revealed a survival advantage for patients receiving TPN. Indeed, in Shamberger's study, there is a suggestion that the tumor-free interval following treatment of lymphoma may be shorter in patients receiving TPN. In patients undergoing surgery, however, especially those who are severely malnourished (as revealed in the VA study) or in patients with major procedures such as esophagogastrectomy (as in Muller's study), evidence suggests that TPN is beneficial. In a late follow-up in Muller's study, there was no apparent increase in recurrence, and the survival rate was the same, despite much higher mortality in the non-TPN group. This suggests that any improved survival following operation may have been offset by an increased late recurrence rate, although it is difficult to reach this conclusion. In summary, for patients with cancer, TPN probably nourishes the tumor as well as the host. Nonetheless, in severely malnourished patients, provision of TPN from 5 to 10 days preoperatively may increase survival and decrease morbidity. Overfeeding must be avoided. Future studies will undoubtedly reveal that there are certain nutrients that tumors require, which probably should best be avoided.

Textbook: Pages 117–119 ANSWER: B

44. Glucose overload results in increased CO_2 production. Which of the following statements is true?

A. In patients with respiratory insufficiency, administration of glucose as a principal source of calories is contraindicated.
B. In patients with pulmonary infection and sepsis, calorie support should consist of 95% fat and 5% glucose.
C. In Askanazi's study, increased CO_2 production and difficulty in weaning were associated only with pronounced overfeeding.
D. CO_2 production should be measured in most patients who are supported by respirators in intensive care units and are receiving nutritional support.

DISCUSSION: Few papers have excited as much interest as that by Askanazi, Kinney, and coworkers, which demonstrated that glucose calories given to patients with severe respiratory impairment may result in difficulty in weaning from a respirator. Subsequent research has suggested, however, that this occurs only with severe overfeeding, when the respiratory quotient is greater than 1 and calories are excessive. If one examines the conditions under which Askanazi's patients were studied, these were a group of septic, depleted patients who were taken from almost no nutritional support to a caloric supply of 2.25 times their caloric requirement, most of the calories consisting of glucose. Suffice it to say that, in patients with impaired respiratory function, one should measure VCO_2 and, when VCO_2 is significantly elevated and appears to interfere with weaning, decrease the amount of glucose calories and increase the amount of fat. If one measures or estimates calorie requirements and does not overfeed, lipid can be used for 25% of the caloric requirement and glucose for the remainder, without much fear of excessive CO_2 production.

Textbook: Pages 120–121 ANSWER: C

45. Hepatic abnormalities have been noted in adults since the beginning of hyperalimentation. Which of the following statements is true?

A. Hepatic steatosis is not associated with an overload of glucose.
B. Hepatic steatosis is usually associated with abnormalities in hepatic enzymes.
C. Hyperbilirubinemia is inevitably associated with hepatic steatosis.

D. Abnormalities in the portal insulin-glucagon ratio are thought to be causative of hepatic steatosis in experimental animals.

DISCUSSION: The most common metabolic complication of total parenteral nutrition in adults is hepatic steatosis. Unlike the hepatic abnormalities in children, which may progress to cholestasis, liver damage, and in some cases death, hepatic steatosis, or fatty infiltration of the liver with triglycerides, appears to be a rather benign complication. It may be, but is not necessarily, associated with hepatic enzymatic abnormalities, which usually occur in the first week, peak at the third week, and generally disappear by the sixth week of parenteral nutrition. Abnormalities in the transaminases are most common, with alkaline phosphatase also being elevated, but there is no correlation between the degree of fatty infiltration and enzymatic abnormalities. Fatty infiltration appears to be largely vacuolization with increased storage of triglycerides. Hepatic steatosis is almost always associated with an overload of glucose. Studies in experimental animals have suggested that the portal insulin-glucagon ratio, which is elevated under these circumstances, may be causally related to hepatic steatosis. Insulin is the leading storage enzyme and is responsible for lipogenesis. The presence of insulin inhibits lipolysis. Glucagon, on the other hand, results in the mobilization of hepatic lipid. The liver "sees" the portal vein insulin-glucagon ratio. Excesses of insulin elicited by hypertonic dextrose increase lipid deposition in the liver, whereas glucagon, which is elicited by certain amino acids, results in the mobilization of hepatic lipid.

Textbook: Pages 120–121

ANSWER: D

NOTES

NOTES

NOTES

CHAPTER 3

PERIOPERATIVE MANAGEMENT

1. Which of the following is not associated with increased likelihood of infection after major elective surgery?

A. Age greater than 70 years.
B. Chronic malnutrition.
C. Controlled diabetes mellitus.
D. Long-term steroid use.
E. Infection at a remote body site.

DISCUSSION: Controlled diabetes mellitus has been shown repeatedly not to be associated with increased likelihood of incisional infection provided one avoids operations on body parts that may be ischemic or neuropathic. Uncontrolled diabetes mellitus, such as ketoacidosis, is associated with a dramatic increase in surgical infection. The other parameters noted—age greater than 70 years, chronic malnutrition, regular steroid use, and an infection at a remote body site—are well-recognized adverse predictive factors and are identified in the textbook.

Textbook: Pages 158–160 ANSWER: C

2. Which of the following is not a determinant of a postoperative cardiac complication?

A. Myocardial infarction 4 months previously.
B. Clinical evidence of congestive heart failure in a patient with 8.5 g/dl hemoglobin.
C. Premature atrial or ventricular contractions on electrocardiogram.
D. A harsh aortic systolic murmur.
E. Age greater than 70 years.

DISCUSSION: Clinical evidence of congestive heart failure in a patient with 8.5 g/dl hemoglobin concentration is a misleading sign. Evidence of congestive failure is ordinarily a major risk factor, but in this particular patient the anemia lends itself to correction by preoperative transfusion with packed red blood cells, and often it is found that congestive heart failure and the associated increased risks disappear when the hemoglobin concentration is returned to the 12 g/dl or higher ratio. All other factors are overt signs of increased likelihood of a postoperative cardiac event, the most ominous being a myocardial infarction 4 months preoperatively or the presence of a harsh aortic systolic murmur suggesting the presence of aortic stenosis. Age greater than 70 years and the presence of premature atrial or ventricular contractions on the electrocardiogram are less strong determinants of a postoperative cardiac complication.

Textbook: Page 160 ANSWER: B

3. Rank the five following clinical scenarios in order of greatest likelihood of serious postoperative pulmonary complications.

A. Transabdominal hysterectomy in an obese woman who requires 3 hours of anesthesia time.
B. Right middle lobectomy for bronchogenic cancer in a 65-year-old smoker.
C. Vagotomy and pyloroplasty for chronic duodenal ulcer disease in a 50-year-old man who had chest film findings of old, healed tuberculosis.
D. Right hemicolectomy in an obese 60-year-old smoker.
E. Modified radical mastectomy in a 58-year-old woman who is obese.

DISCUSSION: If one considers the constellation of risk factors for pulmonary complications that is provided in the tables for this chapter of the textbook (see relevant pages at end of discussion), one should readily recognize right middle lobectomy for bronchogenic cancer in a 65-year-old smoker as the highest risk of a clinical situation for the likelihood of serious pulmonary complications. The next in rank may be properly debated between answer D and answer C. Right hemicolectomy is judged to have somewhat greater likelihood of complications because the patient is older, smokes, and is obese, although the procedure may be done through a transverse or lower abdominal incision. Vagotomy and pyloroplasty is viewed as being somewhat less serious because it is an upper abdominal operation on an elective basis in a 50-year-old man whose only abnormalities include old, healed tuberculosis on a chest film. A very low risk of pulmonary complication should follow a transabdominal hysterectomy done through a lower abdominal incision in a woman whose only risk factors are obesity and a 3-hour anesthesia time. The lowest risk probably resides with the 58-year-old woman undergoing modified radical mastectomy, whose only risk factor is obesity. This is particularly true because this operation is conducted on the surface of the body, is associated with relatively little postoperative pain, and provides free and unrestricted respiratory function.

Textbook: Pages 160–161 ANSWERS: In order—B, D, C, A, E

4. Rank the following seven laboratory tests and procedures in terms of their relative value to a 65-year-old woman who is to undergo elective resection of a sigmoid cancer.

A. Carcinoembryonic antigen (CEA).
B. Blood urea nitrogen.
C. Electrocardiogram.
D. Hemoglobin concentration.
E. Serum creatinine.
F. Arterial blood oxygen tension (PaO_2) on room air.
G. Serum sodium concentration.

DISCUSSION: The most important test by far is the electrocardiogram, with its capacity to indicate signs of occult heart disease. The second most important evaluation is the hemoglobin concentration, which in this patient may show an anemia related to chronic alimentary tract blood loss that would require correction prior to safe induction of a general anesthetic. Arterial blood gases vary from individual to individual, depending primarily on smoking habits and age. Accordingly, each older person should have a resting baseline determination prior to operation. Serum creatinine may show evidence of occult renal disease and is substantially more useful than blood urea nitrogen, which is more vulnerable to transient volume changes. CEA is important to know in many patients with cancer with respect to postoperative follow-up because in some cases it may be an early herald of recurrent disease. However, it has little to do with the patient's preoperative assessment in terms of risk and preparation for an elective operation. The presence of liver metastases, for example, can be discovered with significant accuracy by palpation at the time of operation, and an elevated carcinoembryonic antigen in no set of circumstances would lead one to withhold colon resection with its relief of potential obstruction and bleeding. Finally, serum sodium concentration in a 65-year-old woman who is admitted electively for resection of the colon is always normal and would be of least value among these tests.

Textbook: Pages 157–162 ANSWERS: In order—C, D, F, E, B, A, G

5. Most cautery injuries that occur during laparoscopic surgery are not caused by:

A. Insulation breaks in the electrodes.
B. Sparking from the instrument or electrode tip to the bowel.
C. Use of the bipolar electrocautery.
D. Contact between the bowel and an instrument that is in contact with the electrode tip.
E. Inadvertent touching or grasping of tissue while applying current.

DISCUSSION: Bipolar electrocautery is generally considered much safer than monopolar electrocautery during laparoscopic surgery, particularly in areas with multiple structures. The main causes of injury during laparoscopic surgery remain insulation breaks in the electrodes; sparking from the electrode tip to the bowel; direct contact of an instrument with the bowel while the cautery is activated; and inadvertent touching of tissue while the electrocautery is activated. Because the bipolar electrocautery requires grasping of the structure, collateral current dispersion is minimized because only the tissue between the two electrodes is affected.

Textbook: Page 168 ANSWER: C

6. In general, closed-suction drainage should not be used for which one of the following?

A. Drainage following axillary dissection.
B. Routine operations in the head and neck.
C. Following cholecystectomy for acute cholecystitis.
D. In the subcutaneous tissue of large skin flaps.
E. Abscess drainage for necrotizing pancreatitis.

DISCUSSION: Open-suction drainage should typically be used for drainage of grossly infected fields like that of necrotizing pancreatitis. The Surgical Infection Society has provided guidelines for the usage of surgical drainage. When necessary, closed-suction drainage should be used for clean and clean-contaminated operations. Once a significant infection or abscess has occurred, the use of open-suction drainage (e.g., Davol catheter) is preferred.

Textbook: Page 169 ANSWER: E

7. Which of the following statements is true regarding isoflurane in comparison with halothane?

A. Isoflurane is associated with smoother inhalational induction.
B. Isoflurane produces greater sensitization to the arrhythmogenic effects of catecholamines.
C. Isoflurane has greater potency, as reflected in a lower minimal alveolar concentration.
D. Isoflurane is associated with more rapid emergence.
E. Isoflurane increases bronchoconstriction, whereas halothane decreases bronchoconstriction.

DISCUSSION: Isoflurane is associated with more rapid emergence, as would be predicted from the fact that it has a lower blood-gas solubility coefficient than halothane. Isoflurane is unsuitable for inhalational induction because the vapor is irritating. Halothane produces much greater sensitization to the arrhythmogenic effects of epinephrine. Isoflurane is a less potent anesthetic than halothane, but is about equally effective as a bronchodilator.

Textbook: Pages 258–259 ANSWER: D

8. Which of the following drugs is useful as a premedicant because of its potent amnesic effects?

A. Glycopyrrolate.
B. Etomidate.
C. Midazolam.
D. Ketamine.
E. Thiopental.

DISCUSSION: Glycopyrrolate is an anticholinergic that is used to reduce oropharyngeal secretions and antagonize the cholinergic effects of agents used to reverse neuromuscular blockers. Etomidate, ketamine, and thiopental are intravenous induction agents that are unsuitable for premedication.

Textbook: Page 260 ANSWER: C

9. Which of the following statements most accurately describes the differences between subarachnoid block and epidural block?

A. Subarachnoid block is associated with a more rapid onset of hypotension.
B. Subarachnoid block is associated with greater risk of systemic local anesthetic toxicity.
C. Subarachnoid block is associated with a lower risk of headache after lumbar puncture.
D. Subarachnoid block should not be performed with a mixture of local anesthetic and opioids.
E. Subarachnoid block is associated with a small risk of cardiac arrest from which resuscitation is uncomplicated.

DISCUSSION: Subarachnoid block has a more rapid onset of action than epidural anesthesia and is associated with a more rapid onset of hypotension. Because the dose of local anesthetic is much lower, subarachnoid block is associated with minimal risk of systemic local anesthetic toxicity. Because the epidural needle does not penetrate the dura, the risk of headache after lumbar puncture is negligible unless the dura is inadvertently punctured. Opioids can be added to either subarachnoid or epidural block. If cardiac arrest occurs with subarachnoid block, resuscitation is difficult and requires high doses of epinephrine.

Textbook: Pages 276–278 ANSWER: A

10. Essential monitors for all anesthetics include which of the following ?

A. Direct arterial pressure.
B. Transcutaneous PO_2.
C. Bioimpedance cardiac output.
D. Body temperature.
E. Anesthetic depth (bispectral index).

DISCUSSION: The only essential monitor in the list is body temperature. Each of the others could be used in some cases at the discretion of the anesthesiologist, but none is a standard of care.

Textbook: Pages 264–265 ANSWER: D

11. Which of the following is useful in overcoming airway obstruction during mask ventilation of an anesthetized patient?

A. Flexing the neck at the atlanto-occipital joint.
B. Trendelenburg position.
C. Displacing the mandible anteriorly.
D. Occluding the nares bilaterally.
E. Vigorous painful stimulation.

DISCUSSION: In an anesthetized patient who develops an obstructed airway due to soft tissue relaxation, effective maneuvers include neck *extension* at the atlanto-occipital joint, chin lift, and anterior displacement of the mandible. The other maneuvers would be ineffective.

Textbook: Page 272 ANSWER: C

12. Which of the following statements is accurate regarding preoperative cardiac evaluation?

A. Elderly patients undergoing cataract surgery require preoperative stress testing.
B. Patients who require major vascular surgery should undergo cardiac catheterization before scheduling the vascular procedure.
C. Patients can be stratified for the need for cardiac evaluation based on symptoms and the magnitude of the anticipated surgery.
D. Patients with previous myocardial revascularization are at high risk for perioperative myocardial infarction.
E. Ambulatory electrocardiography is sensitive and specific for the identification of patients at high perioperative risk.

DISCUSSION: Available data suggest that preoperative cardiac evaluation should be based on the patient's symptoms and on the magnitude of the expected surgery. In general, the trend is toward less frequent formal cardiac evaluation. Patients with previous myocardial infarction are at less risk for perioperative myocardial infarction than patients with medically managed angina. Ambulatory electrocardiography is less accurate than dipyridamole thallium scanning.

Textbook: Pages 267–269 ANSWER: C

13. In choosing among the various possibilities for induction of anesthesia, which of the following statements is accurate?

A. Most children under the age of 6 prefer an intravenous induction.
B. Rapid-sequence induction is indicated for patients who have recently eaten and require emergency surgery.
C. Intubation while awake is an obsolete procedure.
D. Mask induction is preferable for general anesthesia for cesarean section.
E. Patients recover from succinylcholine-induced muscle relaxation before becoming hypoxic.

DISCUSSION: Most young children prefer an inhalational induction because they fear needles. Awake intubation remains appropriate for certain patients, particularly those who are expected to be difficult to intubate. Mask induction is contraindicated in cesarean section. Succinylcholine, although short acting, produces muscle relaxation that persists until most unventilated patients have become hypoxic. Rapid-sequence intubation is the preferred approach to patients who have recently eaten and require general anesthesia for emergency surgery.

Textbook: Page 272 ANSWER: B

14. Which of the following statements is accurate regarding local anesthetic toxicity?

A. The earliest symptoms are referable to the central nervous system.
B. At the first sign of local anesthetic toxicity, succinylcholine should be given.
C. When local anesthetics are used for regional block, adding epinephrine decreases the toxic dose.
D. Bupivacaine is the least toxic of currently used local anesthetics.
E. Ester-type local anesthetic agents are more toxic than amide agents because of slow metabolism.

DISCUSSION: Central nervous system symptoms generally precede cardiovascular signs. Succinylcholine is useful for patients who develop seizures secondary to local anesthetic toxicity and who cannot be adequately ventilated as a consequence of seizures. Adding epinephrine increases the toxic dose. Bupivacaine is one of the more toxic local anesthetics. Ester-type local anesthetics are more rapidly metabolized in the plasma and are generally less toxic.

Textbook: Page 262 ANSWER: A

15. Which of the following problems is commonly recognized in the postanesthesia care unit?

A. Delirium.
B. Emesis.
C. Hypoxemia.
D. Hypertension.
E. All of the above.

DISCUSSION: All of the above problems are common in the interval immediately following anesthesia.

Textbook: Pages 278–280 ANSWER: E

16. A 62-year-old man cuts his hand on a broken soft-drink bottle at a family picnic. He has a history of a full tetanus immunization as a child, and his last tetanus toxoid booster was 14 years ago. The proper treatment for him is appropriate local wound care and:

A. Tetanus and diphtheria toxoid (Td) injection.
B. Tetanus immune globulin (TIG) infiltrated into the tissues around the wound and Td.
C. Td and scheduling for additional boosters 1 and 6 months later.
D. Prophylactic antibiotics started immediately and Td.
E. Prophylactic antibiotics started immediately, Td, and TIG injected into the other arm from that used to give Td.

DISCUSSION: TIG is needed only for dirty wounds in patients who have not previously been vaccinated against tetanus. A patient who has had a full initial series needs only to have Td given if the last booster was more than 5 years previously. All adults should have a booster every 10 years, whether or not they suffer an injury. An adult who has not had a full initial series should receive the booster and then be scheduled to complete the series.

Textbook: Pages 174–175 ANSWER: A

17. Preoperative prophylactic antibiotics are recommended for an operation on the stomach in all of the following circumstances except:

A. Gastric outlet obstruction.
B. Gastric cancer.
C. Nissen fundoplication.
D. Gastric ulcer.
E. Gastric restriction procedure for treatment of morbid obesity.

DISCUSSION: Antibiotics are not indicated for a Nissen fundoplication, because they do not enter the lumen of the stomach and thus do not expose the wound to a high risk of bacterial contamination. Even when the stomach is entered, if the patient has normal or increased acid production, bacterial counts are very low and prophylactic antibiotics are not required. With obstruction, gastric cancer, and gastric ulcer, gastric bacterial counts are increased and antibiotics are recommended. Although bacterial counts may or may not be elevated in patients with morbid obesity, excessive weight increases the risk of infection and a controlled trial has shown that prophylactic antibiotics lower the rate of postoperative infection.

Textbook: Page 175 ANSWER: C

18. All of the following are accepted principles for the effective use of prophylactic antibiotics to prevent postoperative infection at the surgical site except:

A. Antibiotics should be administered before the operation is initiated.
B. Antibiotics should be given to maintain therapeutic levels in tissues for the duration of the operation.
C. Cefazolin is the prophylactic antibiotic of choice for an appendectomy.
D. Prophylactic antibiotics should be discontinued within 12 hours after the operation, and in many cases at the end of the procedure.
E. The dose of prophylactic antibiotic used should always be at least as high as the usual therapeutic dose for the drug.

DISCUSSION: An appendectomy involves exposure to colonic bacteria with the probability that *Bacteroides fragilis* will be encountered. Cefazolin, which is appropriate for upper abdominal procedures and those that do not enter the gastrointestinal tract, does not have activity against *B. fragilis*. An appropriate antibiotic following appendectomy would be cefotetan or cefoxitin.

Textbook: Pages 175–176 ANSWER: C

19. Which one of the following statements regarding surgical infections is true?

A. A surgical infection always requires a procedure in the operating room for resolution.

B. A suspected intra-abdominal surgical infection should be treated as soon as possible by high-dose, broad-spectrum antibiotics until a definitive diagnosis can be made.
C. Usually *one* bacterial species is responsible for a serious surgical infection.
D. A postoperative surgical site (wound) infection requires a procedure to achieve resolution.
E. The bacteria responsible for surgical infections usually cause the infection because of special virulence characteristics that allow them to invade the tissues and proliferate.

DISCUSSION: A wound infection needs to be opened for resolution. This may be done in the operating room but is usually accomplished by simply removing the skin sutures or staples and allowing the wound to open and then pursuing a regimen of dressing changes. Not all surgical infections need to be opened in the operating room; however, a postoperative surgical site infection requires a procedure to achieve resolution. A suspected intra-abdominal surgical infection should not be treated as soon as possible because giving antibiotics before making the diagnosis risks delaying the diagnosis and does not cure the infection unless the appropriate procedure is also performed. Most surgical infections are mixed, involving more than one bacterial species, and derive from the endogenous flora where the procedure was performed. The bacteria that cause surgical infections usually do not possess special virulence. Instead, they gain access to the site of infection because of injury to an epithelial surface by trauma, operation, or disease.

Textbook: Page 179 ANSWER: D

20. Signs found in a soft tissue infection indicating that operative exploration and débridement are needed include all except:

A. Very high fever and high white blood cell (WBC) count.
B. Skin necrosis.
C. Crepitus.
D. Bullae.
E. Edema in excess of local signs of infection.

DISCUSSION: Many nonsurgical soft tissue infections are accompanied by a high fever and high WBC count, although this is also common in surgical infections. The four other signs listed commonly denote a necrotizing soft tissue infection that requires operative débridement.

Textbook: Pages 176–178 ANSWER: A

21. Which of the following statements about intra-abdominal infection is not true?

A. Bacterial flora are usually mixed, including both aerobic and anaerobic species.
B. Laparotomy is not required for effective treatment in all cases.
C. Approximately one case in four requires a second procedure to ensure resolution of the infection.
D. Antibiotic therapy must be continued for 10 days to resolve the infection.
E. Initially the choice of antibiotic must be empirical.

DISCUSSION: Many intra-abdominal abscesses can be treated by radiologically guided placement of percutaneous drains instead of laparotomy, and antibiotics need be continued only until the patient has demonstrated a favorable clinical response and has maintained a normal temperature for 24 to 48 hours. Statements A, B, C, and E are true.

Textbook: Page 178 ANSWER: D

22. The principal host target cells of human immunodeficiency virus (HIV) infection that result in profound immunosuppression of the infected patient are:

A. Monocytes.
B. Neutrophils.
C. Kupffer cells.
D. $CD4^+$ lymphocytes.
E. $CD8^+$ lymphocytes.

DISCUSSION: $CD4^+$ lymphocytes, also referred to as T-helper cells, are the primary target of HIV. This results in a relative excess of the $CD8^+$ lymphocyte, which has traditionally been referred to as the T-suppressor cell. The cells of the human inflammatory response and of the reticuloendothelial system are not affected as a primary cell population.

Textbook: Page 190 ANSWER: D

23. Perforation of the gastrointestinal tract in a patient with acquired immunodeficiency syndrome (AIDS), which results in clinical findings of acute peritonitis, is most likely to be:

A. Perforated intestine by cytomegalovirus (CMV) infection.
B. Perforated appendix.
C. Perforated peptic ulcer.
D. Perforated gastric lymphoma.
E. Perforated diverticulitis.

DISCUSSION: Perforated appendicitis is at least as common in the AIDS patient as in the population in general. That makes it the most common cause of peritonitis in the AIDS patient. Although CMV infection is more common in the AIDS patient, intestinal perforation by CMV is still uncommon. Other causes do exist in the AIDS patient but remain much less common than perforated appendix.

Textbook: Page 191 ANSWER: B

24. Which malignancy is most commonly identified as a complication of immunosuppression in the liver transplant patient?

A. Kaposi's sarcoma.
B. Hypernephroma.
C. Squamous carcinoma of the anus.
D. Non-Hodgkin's lymphoma.
E. Bile duct cancer.

DISCUSSION: Lymphomas are the most common malignancy associated with immunosuppression in the liver transplant patient. Skin cancers are most common among kidney transplant cancers. Other cancers are seen in somewhat higher frequencies, but lymphoma is the most common for the liver transplant patient.

Textbook: Pages 193–194 ANSWER: D

25. Which of the following endogenously produced protein signals is not anti-inflammatory?

A. Interleukin-1 (IL-1).
B. IL-4.
C. IL-10.
D. IL-13.
E. Cortisol.

DISCUSSION: IL-1 is a pro-inflammatory cytokine that has endogenous pyrogen activity among other functions. IL-4, IL-10, and IL-13 are counterinflammatory cytokines. Cortisol is the endogenous glucocorticoid steroid from the adrenal gland that has immunosuppressive effects when produced in large quantities during the acute stress response.

Textbook: Pages 28–29 ANSWER: A

26. Immunosuppression due to blood transfusion is secondary to:

A. Shock due to blood loss.
B. The severity of injury.
C. Neutropenia.
D. Depletion of plasma globulins.
E. Unknown.

DISCUSSION: Blood transfusion appears to have immunosuppressive effects, although the severity of the immunosuppression remains debated. The immunosuppressive effects of transfusion are independent of hypotension and the severity of injury. Depletion of blood components with the bleeding and blood replacement process are not responsible for this observation. The specific mechanism of transfusion-associated immunosuppression remains undefined.

Textbook: Page 195 ANSWER: E

27. What organ is likely to be injured when gaining access to the peritoneal cavity for laparoscopic surgery?

A. Transverse colon.
B. Small intestine.
C. Iliac vein.
D. Urinary bladder.

DISCUSSION: The small intestine is the organ that is most likely to be injured when getting access to the peritoneal cavity. The small intestine is injured more frequently than the other organs mentioned because it lies immediately below the umbilicus and occupies the majority of the abdomen. Each of the other organs mentioned is at a lower risk for injury during peritoneal access procedures.

Textbook: Page 300 ANSWER: B

28. Which one of the following statements is most accurate when describing laparoscopy in patients with coexisting cardiovascular disease?

A. End-tidal CO_2 monitoring adequately reflects systemic hypercarbia.
B. Due to a decrease in cardiac output, laparoscopy should always be avoided in these patients.
C. Carbon dioxide pneumoperitoneum causes a decrease in cardiac output that may be poorly tolerated in patients with cardiovascular disease; therefore, careful anesthetic management is important.
D. Central venous pressure is decreased in conjunction with an increase in mean arterial pressure.

DISCUSSION: Pneumoperitoneum causes a decrease in cardiac output. This decrease can have a detrimental effect on patients with existing cardiovascular disease if not monitored and regulated properly. Untoward cardiac events during laparoscopy can be avoided through careful anesthetic management, which calls for invasive cardiac monitoring in patients with cardiovascular disease.

Textbook: Page 294 ANSWER: C

29. Which of the following is most accurate when describing the effects of pneumoperitoneum on the immune response?

A. Systemic immunity is impaired as a result of carbon dioxide (CO_2) pneumoperitoneum.
B. Delayed-type hypersensitivity (DTH) is impaired during and following CO_2 pneumoperitoneum.
C. CO_2 pneumoperitoneum impairs the intra-abdominal local immune response.
D. Presently, a vaccination against the untoward effect of CO_2 pneumoperitoneum is recommended prior to all elective laparoscopic operations.

DISCUSSION: Several laboratories have now shown that systemic immunity is better preserved during CO_2 pneumoperitoneum compared with laparotomy. However, recently the importance of local intraperitoneal immunity during laparoscopy has been recognized. CO_2 pneumoperitoneum causes localized peritoneal acidemia and a decrease in local immunity.

Textbook: Pages 295–297 ANSWER: C

30. Which of the following statements regarding the complications seen with video-assisted thoracic surgery (VATS) is true?

A. The high complication rate for VATS has limited its overall application by thoracic surgeons.
B. The hospital mortality rate for VATS patients is 30 to 40%.
C. The most commonly reported complication following VATS is persistent bleeding.

D. The most commonly reported complication following VATS is a persistent lung air leak.

DISCUSSION: There is a very low hospital mortality rate following VATS. The most commonly reported complication following VATS is a persistent air leak.
Textbook: Page 308 ANSWER: D

31. Which of the following statements regarding the postoperative course of patients undergoing video-assisted thoracic surgery (VATS) is true?

A. On postoperative day 3, there is no difference in the decrease of preoperative pulmonary function in patients undergoing VATS compared to those undergoing thoracotomy.
B. There is no clinical evidence that patients undergoing VATS are discharged sooner than patients undergoing open thoracotomies (the conventional procedure).
C. Patients report improved cosmesis following thoracotomy as compared with VATS.
D. Patients report less pain following VATS compared with thoracotomy.

DISCUSSION: There is a decrease in pulmonary function in patients undergoing VATS in comparison with similar patients undergoing open thoracotomy. Additionally, there is clear evidence that patients undergoing VATS can be discharged from the hospital sooner than their cohorts undergoing open conventional thoracotomies. Finally, when given postoperative questionnaires, patients undergoing VATS reported less postoperative pain compared with similar groups of patients who had undergone traditional thoracotomy.
Textbook: Page 307 ANSWER: D

NOTES

NOTES

NOTES

CHAPTER 4

SURGICAL COMPLICATIONS

1. Which of the following are mechanisms for heat loss that contribute to the development of hypothermia?

A. Radiation.
B. Conduction.
C. Evaporation.
D. Respiration.
E. Convection.
F. All of the above.

DISCUSSION: There are five basic mechanisms for heat loss: radiation (loss of body heat to a cool environment), conduction (direct contact of the body to cooler materials), evaporation (heat loss with evaporated water vapor), respiration (heat loss on exhalation of warmed air), and convection (cool air moves across the warmer body with net loss of heat). In normal circumstances, thermoregulation effectively compensates for these heat losses.

Textbook: Page 204 ANSWER: F

2. Which of the following is required to definitively make a diagnosis of malignant hyperthermia?

A. Administration of an epidural anesthetic.
B. Tachycardia.
C. Cyanosis.
D. Muscle biopsy.
E. Muscle rigidity.
F. Metabolic acidosis.

DISCUSSION: Muscle biopsy is required to confirm the diagnosis of malignant hyperthermia (MH), but the majority of patients have an elevated serum creatinine phosphokinase level. The disorder usually presents within 30 minutes after the administration of anesthetic agents and includes high fever, tachycardia, rigidity, and cyanosis. Hyperkalemia, hypercalcemia, and metabolic acidosis are also associated findings. Treatment includes active cooling of the patient, administration of dantrolene to block the release of calcium from the sarcoplasmic reticulum, and correction of the noted serum electrolyte and acid-base abnormalities. Other types of anesthesia and resuscitation situations can bring about these various metabolic abnormalities and are not diagnostic in and of themselves for MH. A careful preoperative history should note whether the patient or any family members have experienced malignant hyperthermia.

Textbook: Page 205 ANSWER: D

3. Which of the following is not required for the clinical diagnosis of pneumonia?

A. Decreased breath sounds.
B. Temperature that is usually higher than 38.5°C.
C. Pleuritic chest pain with coughing.
D. Elevated peripheral white blood cell count.
E. Chest x-ray infiltrate(s).
F. Positive microbiology cultures from an adequate sputum sample.

DISCUSSION: The patient with atelectasis will have a low-grade temperature and decreased breath sounds in the lower lung fields but may not appear to have significant difficulty breathing. A chest x-ray may show only areas of partial collapse and may not be specific otherwise. The diagnosis of pneumonia still rests on the presence of fever, an elevated white blood cell count, the presence of infiltrates on chest x-ray, and the production of thick secretions that yield positive microbiology cultures. These patients often appear toxic and are not able to take deep breaths or cough effectively. On the severe end of the spectrum, patients may be in full respiratory failure with rapid respirations, increased work of breathing, and significantly low oxygen saturation despite supplemental oxygen. Pleuritic chest pain is not usually diagnostic of pneumonia.

Textbook: Pages 205–206 ANSWER: C

4. The adult respiratory distress syndrome (ARDS) does not have which of the following two items that are required for making the diagnosis of acute lung injury (ALI)?

A. Pulmonary capillary wedge pressure <20 mm Hg.
B. PaO_2/FIO_2 ratio of <300.
C. PaO_2/FIO_2 ratio of <200.
D. Bilateral infiltrates on chest x-ray.
E. An acute change in lung function.

DISCUSSION: In response to several stimuli, the various immune mediator cascades create a typical pathophysiologic inflammatory response in (ALI) and ARDS that leads to accumulation of fluid in the extravascular and intra-alveolar spaces of the lung parenchyma. The gas exchange abnormalities are similar and are characterized by ventilation-perfusion mismatching that result in pulmonary shunting and increased ventilatory dead space. The most widely accepted definition of ARDS is: (1) an acute change in

lung function, (2) bilateral infiltrates on chest x-ray, (3) a pulmonary capillary wedge pressure less than 20 mm Hg and no evidence for congestive heart failure, and (4) a PaO_2/FIO_2 ratio of less than 200. The same criteria are accepted for ALI except that the PaO_2/FIO_2 ratio is set at less than 300. Hydrostatic pulmonary edema is related most commonly to congestive heart failure or vascular fluid overload and the patient often has a pulmonary capillary wedge pressure higher than 20 mm Hg.
Textbook: Page 207 ANSWER: B

5. What is the expected myocardial reinfarction rate for patients undergoing noncardiac surgery following a recent acute myocardial infarction (AMI)?

A. No difference compared with other myocardial infarction patients.
B. 27% at less than 3 months; 10% at 3 to 6 months; 5% at more than 6 months.
C. 20% in the first 6 months and then similar to other myocardial infarction patients.
D. 15% at less than 3 months; 10% at 3 to 6 months; 5% at more than 6 months.
E. 50% at less than 3 months; 25% at 3 to 6 months; 15% at more than 6 months.
F. None of the above.

DISCUSSION: The mortality rate from a perioperative AMI can be as high as 50 to 90% and the vast majority of deaths occur in the first 48 hours after surgery. This compares dramatically to the general mortality of 12% for AMI in patients that do not have a surgical procedure. Shock in the perioperative period (hypotension sustained for 10 minutes or longer) is the most commonly associated finding in patients that develop a perioperative AMI. For patients with a previous AMI who require surgery, the reinfarction rate is directly correlated to the amount of time since the original AMI. If operated on within 3 months of an AMI, the reinfarction rate is about 27%. This decreases to roughly 10% if the time period after an AMI is 3 to 6 months. Beyond 6 months, the reinfarction rate resembles the general AMI reinfarction rate of 5 to 8%.
Textbook: Page 209 ANSWER: B

6. Components of the syndrome of inappropriate antidiuretic hormone (SIADH) include:

A. Hyponatremia.
B. Hypernatremia.
C. Peripheral edema.
D. Serum hyperosmolality.
E. Hypertension.

DISCUSSION: SIADH occurs when there is an increased production of ADH. This can be secondary to drugs, ADH-producing tumors, and central nervous system disorders. The principal action of ADH is water resorption at the level of the collecting tubules, leading to an expanded intravascular volume and resulting hyponatremia. Patients are normotensive, have no peripheral edema, and a low serum osmolality as well as urine hyperosmolality.
Textbook: Page 214 ANSWER: A

7. The most common cause of a small bowel obstruction is:

A. Hernia.
B. Tumor.
C. Volvulus.
D. Adhesions.
E. Ileocolic intussusception.

DISCUSSION: The most common etiology of a small bowel obstruction is adhesions, especially after pelvic surgery. This is followed by tumors, hernias, and volvulus as causes. A postoperative intussusception can occur in children, but is rare in an adult.
Textbook: Page 215 ANSWER: D

8. An abdominal compartment syndrome produces all of the following except:

A. Acute renal failure.
B. Hypoxia.
C. Intestinal obstruction.
D. Elevated urinary bladder pressure.
E. Hypercarbia.

DISCUSSION: An abdominal compartment syndrome exists when intra-abdominal pressure becomes higher than 15 mm Hg. This is reflected in an elevated urinary bladder pressure. Compression of intra-abdominal contents leads to acute renal failure, and abdominal distention leads to respiratory failure with hypoxia and hypercarbia. Intestinal obstruction is not caused by elevated intra-abdominal pressure.
Textbook: Pages 215–216 ANSWER: C

9. Initial treatment of acute gastrointestinal bleeding includes:

A. H_2-receptor antagonists.
B. Aggressive volume resuscitation.
C. Gastrointestinal endoscopy.
D. Sucralfate.
E. Antibiotics.

DISCUSSION: The initial treatment of gastrointestinal bleeding includes patient stabilization with aggressive volume resuscitation. Endoscopy can provide an etiology for the bleeding and direct site-specific treatment, but should not be performed in an unstable patient. Acid-reducing medications, including H_2-receptor antagonists and antacids, are helpful in the prevention of stress ulceration and in the healing process but do not prevent episodes of bleeding or reduce the need for surgical intervention. Antibiotics do not play a role in therapy for gastrointestinal bleeding.
Textbook: Page 216 ANSWER: B

10. Surgical antibiotic prophylaxis is indicated:

A. In all emergency operations.
B. Wounds classified as clean-contaminated.
C. Wounds classified as contaminated.
D. Wounds classified as dirty-infected.
E. All wounds.

DISCUSSION: Surgical antibiotic prophylaxis is indicated only in clean-contaminated wounds, in which the respiratory, alimentary, genital, or urinary tracts are entered under controlled conditions, and without unusual contamination. Clean wounds and emergency procedures are not candidates for prophylaxis, unless a foreign body (prosthesis) is placed, or the location is at high risk for infection (e.g., intracranial procedures). Contaminated and dirty-infected wounds are treated with empirical antibiotics with adjustments made after culture results are obtained.

Textbook: Page 202 ANSWER: B

11. Postrenal causes of acute renal failure include all of the following except:

A. Ureteral obstruction due to stones.
B. Bladder dysfunction due to nerve injury.
C. Urethral obstruction due to prostatic enlargement.
D. A blocked Foley catheter.
E. Myoglobinuria.

DISCUSSION: Myoglobin obstructs the collecting tubules with the kidney, and is therefore an intrarenal cause of acute renal failure. All others are examples of postrenal causes.

Textbook: Page 211 ANSWER: E

12. Which of the following statements is true?

A. Life expectancy of a patient aged 100 years, who has no comorbid conditions, is 6 months.
B. The proportion of persons aged 65 and older will remain constant over the next 50 years.
C. Age is frequently a risk factor in predicting postoperative morbidity and mortality.
D. Life expectancy for men is 72 years and for women, 78 years.

DISCUSSION: The life expectancy for a healthy centenerian is approximately 2.7 years. The proportion of persons over the age of 65 is expected to double over the next 50 years and comprise at least one quarter of the population. Although age frequently appears as a risk when univariate analysis is used, when multivariate analysis (a more accurate measure of risk) is employed, age frequently falls out as a significant factor. Based on 1991 data, men are expected to live 72 years and women, 78 years.

Textbook: Page 226 ANSWER: D

13. Which of the following statements is false?

A. Systolic cardiac function decreases with age at a constant rate.
B. Predictable decreases in renal function occur with age, and relate specifically to the glomerular filtration rate.
C. Normal white blood cell (WBC) counts are frequently seen in an aged immune system.
D. Both forced vital capacity (FVC) and forced expiratory volume in 1 second (FEV_1) decrease steadily with aging.

DISCUSSION: Although diastolic function of the heart typically decreases with aging, systolic function remains normal. Renal function decreases at a defined rate, and relates to age and weight. Serum creatinine does not change because along with the decreased renal function is a decreased lean body mass. Although there are changes in T-cell function and bone marrow response to immunologic stress, the total WBC count typically remains unchanged in normal individuals. Loss of elastic recoil results in decreased FVC and FEV_1, but only mild increases occur in resting volume and functional residual capacity. After surgery, however, the latter can increase substantially.

Textbook: Pages 228–232 ANSWER: A

14. In which of the following has chronologic age been clearly shown to be a factor in prognosis?

A. Papillary carcinoma of the thyroid.
B. Colorectal surgery.
C. Breast cancer.
D. American Society of Anesthesiology (ASA) classification of risk.

DISCUSSION: For thyroid cancer the AMES (age, metastases, extent, and size) classification of risk has shown that age greater than 41 years in men and greater than 51 years in women is a poor prognostic indicator. It is currently not clear whether breast cancer in elderly patients has a different course than in younger ones, and older patients should be surgically and medically treated the same as younger ones. Although some studies have shown that elderly patients undergoing colorectal surgery are at increased risk, when multivariate analysis is employed, the presence of concomitant disease and emergency procedures correlates with complications and death, not chronologic age. Age is not part of the ASA classification. Comparative studies have in fact shown that age plays a minor role in predicting risk for operative procedures. Other disease processes directly linked to chronologic age are trauma and burns.

Textbook: Pages 616–620 ANSWER: A

15. In emergency surgery for perforated ulcer disease, a patient with preoperative shock, greater than 48 hours of perforation, and significant comorbid cardiac disease has a mortality rate close to:

A. 0%.
B. 25%.
C. 50%.
D. 100%.

DISCUSSION: Multivariate analysis of patient data from Boey and coworkers (Ann Surg 205:22, 1987) has shown that age, amount of soiling, and length of symptoms have no predictive value. The three factors mentioned in the question were predictive. If none of the factors are present, the mortality rate is 0%; if one is present, the mortality rate is 10%; if two are present, the mortality rate is 46%; and if all three are present, the rate approaches 100%. For bleeding ulcer, the presence of an ulcer larger than 1 cm, a 5-unit bleed,

and the presence of comorbid illness are predictive of mortality (Ann Surg 211:411, 1990).
Textbook: Page 237 ANSWER: D

16. Which of the following is true regarding appendicitis in the elderly?
A. Most patients present with classic signs and symptoms of right lower quadrant pain, increased white blood cell count, and fever.
B. Although there are typically delays in presentation to the hospital, the diagnosis is usually made in a timely fashion.
C. Reported rates of perforated appendicitis in the octogenerian are below 50%.
D. Twenty percent of patients present with no abdominal pain.

DISCUSSION: Only 50% of elderly persons with acute appendicitis present with classic signs and symptoms. Upward of 20% of patients present with no abdominal pain. Although many present late to the hospital, the diagnosis is frequently delayed because of confusion in the diagnosis. Newer tests, such as helical computed tomography scanning, may help make the diagnosis earlier.
Textbook: Page 240 ANSWER: D

17. In the elderly patient with suspected biliary disease, which of the following statements is false?
A. The rate of gallstones is as high as 30 to 40% of persons over the age of 80 years.
B. There is an increased incidence of common bile duct stones in persons undergoing cholecystectomy.
C. Gallbladder motility is typically normal.
D. The conversion rate from laparoscopic cholecystectomy to open procedures is higher than in younger groups.

DISCUSSION: As noted for appendicitis, elderly persons with biliary disease usually present later, and only 50% have classic symptoms. The net result is that more severe disease is encountered at surgery, including common bile duct stones, gangrene, and inflammation. This leads to higher conversion rates. Decreased cholesterol metabolism by the liver occurs with aging, resulting in higher biliary cholesterol and lithogenicity of bile. Similarly, decreased gallbladder motility parallels aging, resulting in stasis and gallstone formation.
Textbook: Pages 238–239 ANSWER: D

18. Midazolam results in all of the following except:
A. Respiratory depression.
B. Hypotension.
C. Sedation.
D. Analgesia.
E. Amnesia.

DISCUSSION: Midazolam is a benzodiazepine with strong sedative and amnestic properties. Side effects include respiratory and cardiovascular depression. The drug does not provide any appreciable analgesia.
Textbook: Pages 289–290 ANSWER: D

19. The narcotic of choice for bolus intrathecal administration for spinal anesthesia is:
A. Morphine.
B. Fentanyl.
C. Alfentanyl.
D. Hydrocodone.
E. Oxycodone.

DISCUSSION: When injecting a narcotic for spinal analgesia, the optimal properties are long duration of action. Fentanyl and alfentanyl are so lipid soluble that their duration of action is very short compared with morphine. Both hydrocodone and oxycodone are oral drugs and contraindicated for intrathecal injection.
Textbook: Pages 285–286 ANSWER: A

20. On completion of an inguinal herniorrhaphy under general anesthesia, the surgeon wishes to infiltrate local anesthesia into the operative field to provide postoperative analgesia for the patient. The best choice of drug and amount is:
A. 500 mg of 1% lidocaine with epinephrine.
B. 100 mg of 1% lidocaine with epinephrine.
C. 200 mg of 0.25% bupivacaine with epinephrine.
D. 500 mg of 0.25% bupivacaine with epinephrine.
E. 500 mg of 1% lidocaine without epinephrine.

DISCUSSION: When infusing local anesthetic for postoperative analgesia, a longer-acting medication such as bupivacaine is preferred. The maximum recommended dose of the drug if given with epinephrine is 225 mg, so 500 mg would be an overdose and potentially result in convulsions and respiratory depression.
Textbook: Pages 262–263, 278 ANSWER: C

21. Important actions the surgeon can perform preoperatively to help ensure good pain control in the postoperative period include all of the following except:
A. Educate the patient regarding the incision site and the area that will be painful postoperatively.
B. Prescribe both a mechanical and antibiotic bowel prep.
C. Choose a minimally invasive approach to perform the operation.
D. Discuss with the patient the plan for postoperative activity.
E. Arrange a preoperative consultation with the anesthesiologist for consideration of an epidural catheter postoperatively.

DISCUSSION: All of the above measures except the bowel prep are likely to both educate and reassure the patient of what to expect in the postoperative period. Knowing that the issues of pain and pain control are being addressed preoperatively is reassuring to the patient. Choosing a minimally invasive approach to perform the operation is associated with a decrease in postoperative pain for most operations.
Textbook: Page 284 ANSWER: B

22. During conscious sedation, the patient should be expected to:

A. Answer questions without slurred speech.
B. Maintain oxygen saturation of over 97%.
C. Become sedated with 50 μg of fentanyl.
D. Require flumazenil in 25% of cases.
E. Guard and maintain a patent airway.

DISCUSSION: During conscious sedation, the patient should be expected to maintain a patent airway; otherwise, the sedation is considered excessive and defined as a level of anesthesia. Appropriate conscious sedation rarely requires reversal with flumazenil, and patients may experience slurring of speech and mild oxygen desaturation to 90%, at which point supplemental oxygen is placed. In normal circumstances, 50 μg of fentanyl alone will not provide adequate sedation for procedures requiring conscious sedation.

Textbook: Page 289 ANSWER: E

23. The site of action of systemic opioids on nociceptive transmission is:

A. Unmyelinated type C peripheral nerve fibers.
B. Inhibitory interneurons of the spinal tract projecting on spinal interneurons.
C. Neurons in the spinothalamic tract or their thalamocortical projections.
D. The primary afferent nociceptors.
E. Sympathetic efferent fibers.

DISCUSSION: Nociceptive transmission is affected by systemic opioids only in the central nervous system itself. These areas would include the spinothalamic tracts, their thalamocortical projections, and the cortex itself. Epidural opioids may influence transmission at the spinal neuron level. Opioids are not felt to act on peripheral afferent nerves or primary afferent nociceptors. Sympathetic afferent fibers are not involved in nociceptive transmission.

Textbook: Pages 286–289 ANSWER: C

24. Nonsteroidal anti-inflammatory drugs (NSAIDs) are felt to cause analgesia due to:

A. Their ability to cross the blood-brain barrier.
B. Action at hydroxy-tryptamine (HT)–4 receptors to block serotonin release.
C. Action at mu-2 opioid receptors.
D. Inhibition of cyclooxygenase and prostaglandin production.
E. Inhibition of macrophage release of cytokines.

DISCUSSION: NSAIDs as a group provide analgesia through inhibition of the inflammatory response, and have their direct action on cyclooxygenase, thereby inhibiting prostaglandin production. None of the other answers are correct.

Textbook: Page 288 ANSWER: D

25. Which of the following regarding morbid obesity is incorrect?

A. Morbidly obese patients who are 20 to 40 years of age may experience a 12-fold reduction in life expectancy in comparison with their age-matched controls.
B. Morbid obesity is defined as a body mass index (BMI) greater than 40 kg/m^2 or a BMI greater than 35 kg/m^2 with concomitant obesity-related morbidities.
C. Type II noninsulin-dependent diabetes can be corrected with successful weight loss in the majority of morbidly obese patients, but hypertension rarely improves.
D. Morbidly obese women have an increased cancer mortality rate from endometrial, uterine cervix, ovarian, and breast cancer.

DISCUSSION: Obese patients are at increased risk of illness from coronary artery disease, hypertension, Type II diabetes, respiratory insufficiency, venous stasis or thromboembolic disease, debilitating arthritis of weight-bearing joints, and depression, as well as uterine, ovarian, colon, breast, and prostate cancer. Life expectancy can be reduced 12-fold for morbidly obese patients who are 20 to 40 years of age compared with age-matched controls. Successful bariatric surgery can eliminate many of the obesity-related morbidities. Successful weight loss after Roux-en-Y gastric bypass should eliminate Type II noninsulin-dependent diabetes in 90% of patients and hypertension in 80% of patients.

Textbook: Page 248 ANSWER: C

26. With regard to the genetics of human obesity, which of the following is correct?

A. The protein encoded by the obesity gene *(ob)* is leptin.
B. Elevated blood levels of leptin have been associated with an increased percentage of fat, an increased body mass index (BMI), and insulin resistance.
C. A genetic mutation in the coding for a leptin receptor gene has been identified only in mice.
D. Genetic therapies manipulating the glucocorticoid receptor gene, the β_3-adrenergic receptor gene, and the sulfonylurea receptor gene represent potential treatment strategies for obesity.
E. All of the above.

DISCUSSION: In 1994, Zhang reported that hereditary obesity in mice was due to the mutated *ob* gene which encodes the protein leptin. Leptin is a 16-kD glycoprotein secreted primarily from adipose tissue that is thought to be a primary regulator of metabolism by acting as a satiety signaler and impairing insulin-mediated glucose uptake in skeletal muscle, stimulating lipogenic enzymes in adipocytes, and altering hypothalamic-pituitary-adrenal balance. Elevated leptin blood levels in humans are associated with an increased percentage of body fat, BMI, and the insulin resistance syndrome, characterized by high blood pressure, low levels of high-density lipoprotein cholesterol, and elevated fasting insulin levels. The human obesity gene and the leptin receptor gene have been cloned, and members of families with a mutation in the coding sequence of the leptin-receptor gene have been identified. Other genetic mutations have been identified, such as the glucocorticoid receptor gene responsible for glucocorticoid promotion of visceral fat accumulation, the β_3-adrenergic receptor responsible for the catecholamine effect on energy metabolism, and the sulfonylurea receptor gene responsible for glucose-stimulated insulin secretion.

Textbook: Page 248 ANSWER: E

27. With regard to Roux-en-Y gastric bypass, which of the following statements is correct?

A. In prospective, randomized trials, vertical banded gastroplasty has been more successful than Roux-en-Y gastric bypass in the long-term maintenance of weight loss.
B. Roux limbs up to 150 cm in length have been used successfully for long-term weight loss in patients with super obesity (BMI greater than 50 kg/m²).
C. The gastric pouch should be 100 to 150 ml and the gastrojejunostomy outlet 1.2 cm in diameter.
D. Long-term control of Type II noninsulin-dependent diabetes can be expected postoperatively in about 10% of patients after a Roux-en-Y gastric bypass.

DISCUSSION: The isolated gastric pouch for a Roux-en-Y gastric bypass is constructed to hold only 15 to 30 ml. The Roux limb is prepared by transecting the jejunum approximately 60 cm distal to the ligament of Treitz. The outlet from the gastric pouch to the Roux limb (gastrojejunostomy) should be 1.2 cm in diameter. The enteroenterostomy (biliary limb to Roux limb) is constructed 60 cm distal to the gastrojejunostomy. A longer Roux limb increases malabsorption, and Roux limbs of 150 cm have been used successfully in patients with super obesity (BMI greater than 50 kg/m²). Long-term control of adult-onset diabetes is achieved in 90% of patients after Roux-en-Y gastric bypass. Prospective randomized studies comparing vertical banded gastroplasty with gastric bypass demonstrated significantly less weight loss for patients undergoing vertical banded gastroplasty.

Textbook: Page 251 ANSWER: B

28. Which of the following is not a common indication for revision of a vertical banded gastroplasty?

A. Inadequate weight loss.
B. Electrolyte disturbances (i.e., hypocalcemia, hypomagnesemia, hypokalemia) and protein-calorie malnutrition.
C. Staple line dehiscence.
D. Outlet stenosis.

DISCUSSION: Postoperative complications of vertical banded gastroplasty include leak (0.6%), wound infection (1.5%), staple line dehiscence (2 to 7%), outlet stenosis (2.5 to 8.0%), and band erosion (1 to 2%). Revisionary rates for vertical banded gastroplasty are 0.8 to 1.8% per year and approximately 5 to 36% of patients will require reoperation for inadequate weight loss, outlet stenosis, band erosion, or staple line dehiscence. Inadequate weight loss is usually due to a staple line dehiscence or an outlet dilatation. An additional cause of weight loss failure after vertical banded gastroplasty is a change in dietary habits toward high calorie liquids and sweets. Because vertical banded gastroplasty eliminates only the reservoir function of the stomach and does not bypass any part of the gastrointestinal tract, the incidence of malnutrition-related complications are lower than gastric bypass. Stomal ulcers can develop following gastric bypass in two instances: after construction of a large gastric pouch containing acid-secreting cells or after a staple line dehiscence allowing acid reflux.

Textbook: Pages 250–251 ANSWER: B

29. Which of the following metabolic abnormalities or complications is associated with a biliopancreatic bypass?

A. Protein-calorie malnutrition.
B. Hypocalcemia and vitamin D deficiency.
C. Iron deficiency.
D. Folate and vitamin B_{12} deficiency.
E. All of the above.

DISCUSSION: Biliopancreatic bypass combines a subtotal gastrectomy with a Roux-en-Y gastroileal anastomosis and a jejunoileal anastomosis 50 cm proximal to the ileocecal valve to allow absorption of nutrients in the distal 50 cm of the common channel. Complications associated with the procedure are protein malnutrition and malabsorption of vitamins. In order to reduce these complications, the operation was modified to include a duodenal switch, constructed by performing a sleeve gastrectomy instead of subtotal gastrectomy, a Roux-en-Y duodenoileal anastomosis and an ileoileal anastomosis 100 cm proximal to the ileocecal valve. The modifications reduced the incidence of malabsorption. Nevertheless, late complications include marginal ulceration (12%); bone demineralization (6.0%) secondary to calcium and vitamin D deficiencies; protein-calorie malnutrition (15.1%) characterized by hypoalbuminemia, anemia, edema, asthenia, and alopecia; and vitamin B_{12}, iron, and folate deficiencies (5.0%).

Textbook: Pages 252–253 ANSWER: E

NOTES

NOTES

CHAPTER 5

TRAUMA AND CRITICAL CARE

1. A 42-year-old man is admitted following a motor vehicle crash. He was restrained with lap belt and shoulder restraint and is complaining of sternal pain. Physical examination is remarkable for chest wall contusion, but chest x-ray is normal. Appropriate diagnosis of myocardial contusion is best accomplished with:

A. Twelve-lead electrocardiography (ECG).
B. Telemetry.
C. Serial creatine phosphokinase (CPK) isoenzymes.
D. Cardiac echography.
E. Thallium scan.

DISCUSSION: The diagnosis of blunt myocardial injury is often difficult. A variety of tests have been advocated and evaluated since the 1990s. These include CPK isoenzymes, cardiac echography, thallium scanning, and ECG evaluation. The two most important clinical complications of myocardial contusion are arrythmias and low cardiac output. Both of these complications are relatively infrequent, which makes predicting them by any one test challenging. Of all tests evaluated to date, the electrocardiogram remains the most sensitive and specific test to reliably make the diagnosis of myocardial contusion, particularly a myocardial contusion that may be associated with complications of arrhythmia or low output. In a patient with ECG evidence of myocardial contusion, subsequent monitoring for 12 to 24 hours is the usual treatment. For patients who may have hemodynamically stressful challenges, some would advocate the use of echography to demonstrate dyskinesis and thereby predict a need for advanced monitoring during surgery.

Textbook: Page 329 ANSWER: A

2. A 32-year-old man is admitted following ejection from his vehicle. He is unresponsive, but moves his upper and lower extremities to pain. He has been intubated in the field and arrives hypotensive with diminished breath sounds in the right chest. Blood pressure is 80/60 and abdomen is distended. Initial management should be:

A. Hyperventilation.
B. Needle decompression of the right chest.
C. Immediate diagnostic peritoneal lavage.
D. Placement of right subclavian intravenous filter.
E. Transfusion of type O negative blood.

DISCUSSION: The basic problem with this patient is that he is hypotensive and has several potential etiologies for the hypotension. Although the patient probably has a significant head injury by his presentation, head injury is the least likely cause of the patient's hypotension. The patient also has diminished breath sounds with the assumption of a pneumothorax and a distended abdomen with the presumption of intra-abdominal bleeding. The dilemma here is whether the pneumothorax is a tension pneumothorax that is causing the hypotension, or whether the patient simply has a simple pneumothorax, but is hypotensive due to hypovolemia. The correct sequencing of this dilemma is to decompress the pneumothorax, thereby removing this as a possibility to explain the hypotension and subsequently beginning volume resuscitation. Beginning volume resuscitation in the presence of a tension pneumothorax is unlikely to resolve the patient's problem. Therefore, the only logical answer is needle decompression of the right chest. Although needle decompression is the most rapid way to relieve the pneumothorax, it should be said that one should follow this by a tube thoracostomy. Needle decompression can, at times, be ineffective and is not a long-term management for tension pneumothorax. Tube thoracostomy is the definitive solution.

Textbook: Pages 327–329 ANSWER: B

3. A 32-year-old man is ejected from his motorcycle and presents hypotensive, complaining of abdominal and pelvic pain. Diagnostic peritoneal lavage (DPL) is 115,000 red blood cells (RBC) and pelvic x-ray reveals a large sacral fracture and pelvic diastasis greater than 10 cm. Blood pressure remained 90/50 following 4 units of packed RBC and placement of military antishock trousers (MAST). The next appropriate treatment would be:

A. Laparotomy and control of bleeding, and packing of the pelvic hematoma.
B. Application of external fixation, followed by laparotomy.
C. Angiography and embolization, followed by external fixation.
D. Laparotomy and immediate open reduction and internal fixation of the pelvic fracture.
E. External fixation and tibial traction with transfusion.

DISCUSSION: This patient presents a dilemma between attributing hypotension from bleeding to an intra-abdominal source and a pelvic fracture source. Initial screening for intra-abdominal bleeding in a hypotensive patient may be done by some with ultrasound, but traditionally is done with DPL, as the patient's hemodynamic instability precludes going to a computed tomography scan. If lavage is performed, the traditional threshold for operation has been 100,000 RBC. In the presence of a pelvic fracture, there may be some bleeding intraperitoneally that is due to the pelvic fracture, but more importantly, a modest elevation above 100,000 RBC is not sufficient intra-abdominal bleeding to explain the patient's hypotension. Given the scenario as presented, the DPL of 115,000 is unlikely to be the cause of the patient's major bleeding and hypotension. The patient has a known pelvic fracture. This source is much more likely. When coupled with the fact that the patient has been transfused 4 units of blood, it is then most appropriate to go first to angiography. This would be the best sequence to slow the patient's bleeding.

Textbook: Page 342 ANSWER: C

4. A 25-year-old woman sustains blunt abdominal trauma following a motor vehicle crash. She remains hemodynamically stable and abdominal computed tomography (CT) scan is remarkable for a liver laceration. The best criterion that would indicate failure with nonoperative management would be:

A. Grade III laceration or greater.
B. Greater than 150 ml of intraperitoneal blood.
C. Transfusion of >2 units during the first 12 hours.
D. CT intravenous contrast extravasation.
E. Intrahepatic hematoma >10 cm.

DISCUSSION: Over the past 5 years nonoperative management of liver and spleen injuries has evolved rapidly. Currently, as many as 80 to 90% of low-grade lesions (I, II, and III) are being managed nonoperatively and as many as 50% of more severe lesions (Grades IV and V) are being managed nonoperatively. Specific criteria as contraindications to nonoperative management are not well established. It is clear that most patients who can successfully be managed nonoperatively will require fewer transfusions and have less blood on CT scan; however, many examples of patients being managed with greater than 500 ml of intraperitoneal blood and transfusions greater than 2 units have been reported. The extravasation of contrast material is a universally agreed-on indication of active bleeding and most consider this a criterion not to pursue nonoperative management. The role of angiography in this circumstance is being evaluated, but is not considered a routine step. Until its role is further defined, operative management of patients with CT contrast extravasation should be followed.

Textbook: Pages 336–339 ANSWER: D

5. Six hours after falling from a ladder, a 46-year-old man is transferred to your institution. He responded initially to crystalloid resuscitation and has been stable in transit. He has three left-sided rib fractures and a nondisplaced fracture of the femur. Hemoglobin is 12. A computed tomography (CT) scan of the abdomen shows a Grade III–IV hilar injury of the spleen without vascular extravasation. The most appropriate next step in management is:

A. Immediate angiography and embolization.
B. Treatment of the femoral fracture in less than 12 hours.
C. Admission to the intensive care unit with serial examinations and hemoglobin determinations.
D. Urgent laparotomy with splenorrhaphy or splenectomy.
E. Give Pneumovax and antibiotics prior to splenectomy.

DISCUSSION: This patient is hemodynamically stable, has not required transfusion, has an acceptable hemoglobin, and has no evidence of ongoing bleeding, despite a Grade III–IV splenic laceration. CT scan is known to probably upgrade splenic injuries relative to the actual injury and is only a relative indicator of whether or not a patient will have successful nonoperative management. As such, the patient who is hemodynamically stable and has evidence of splenic laceration is appropriately managed by serial examination, serial hematocrit determinations, with an eye toward ultimately successful nonoperative management. Pre-emptive angiography and urgent laparotomy are not necessary, and Pneumovax and antibiotics would be inappropriate unless the patient went to splenectomy. The need to fix a femur fracture within 12 hours is unfounded, although most agree that fixation within 24 hours is appropriate. Although urgent fixation of fractures is perhaps ultimately always better, in the case in which there is a competing injury that requires observation, there is no urgency to fix the femur fracture. Delaying 12 hours, which is about the amount of time that would be needed to decide about failure of nonoperative management for the spleen, would be a common interval.

Textbook: Pages 339–340 ANSWER: C

6. A 20-year-old man is admitted to the emergency department 15 minutes after being shot in the abdomen. Blood pressure is 110/80 and wounds are noted anteriorly just to the left of the umbilicus and posteriorly to the left of the third lumbar vertebra. During evaluation, the patient's blood pressure falls to 80/0 and heart rate is 160. Appropriate management would be:

A. Resuscitative thoracotomy.
B. Pericardiocentesis.
C. Transfer to the intensive care unit for immediate transfusion.
D. Insertion of pulmonary artery catheter.
E. Immediate celiotomy.

DISCUSSION: This patient presents with a gunshot wound to the abdomen and is hemodynamically stable and then deteriorates. The tract of the bullet is such that it is very *unlikely* that there is chest involvement, and rapid fluid resuscitation and celiotomy would be the most appropriate management. There are those who would advocate for resuscitative thoracotomy prior to celiotomy; however, if the patient can be resuscitated, there is no evidence that this is a superior management strategy. Control of the intra-abdominal aorta with compression is as effective as resuscitative thoracotomy, although this continues to be debated.

Textbook: Pages 1409–1413 ANSWER: E

7. A 37-year-old woman presents 4 hours following a motor vehicle crash with an anterior abdominal wall contusion from the lap belt. The most sensitive diagnostic test to detect perforation would be:

A. Abdominal ultrasound.
B. Diagnostic peritoneal lavage (DPL).
C. Abdominal computed tomography (CT) scan.
D. Gastrografin upper gastrointestinal (GI) x-ray.
E. Serial abdominal examination.

DISCUSSION: This case represents a dilemma of a patient presenting with an anterior abdominal wall contusion from a lap belt and the potential for blunt visceral injury. This remains one of the most challenging diagnostic dilemmas in abdominal trauma and is complicated by a delay in diagnosis in 30 to 50% of reported series. The reason for this remains the relative nonspecificity and insensitivity of the traditional objective evaluation of the abdomen techniques including CT scan, ultrasound, and DPL. Some have advocated routine laparotomy in the presence of an abdominal wall contusion, but with increased use of restraints and the increased frequency of this presenting symptom, routine laparotomy is not appropriate either. CT scan, ultrasound, and DPL each have a false-negative rate associated with this, but of the tests currently available, CT probably has the greatest sensitivity. In a patient presenting 4 hours following injury, the interpretation of DPL and ultrasound will not be as straightforward as in a patient presenting immediately. In this case, a small amount of intra-abdominal bleeding might be misinterpreted by a DPL, and criteria for the use of ultrasound in delayed presentation are not as clearly defined. Serial abdominal examination is part of any management if the initial diagnostic test is negative. The use of an upper GI x-ray with contrast is useful for the detection of retroperitoneal duodenal injury, but with the advent of CT scan and the use of oral contrast, there is no evidence that the traditional upper GI radiograph is any more sensitive.

Textbook: Page 335 ANSWER: C

8. A 23-year-old man sustains a gunshot wound to the abdomen with a large pelvic hematoma in the right pelvis. Exploration reveals bleeding from the bifurcation of the vena cava. Control of bleeding should occur with:

A. Ligation of the iliac veins and vena cava.
B. Packing and re-exploration in 48 hours.
C. Division of the iliac artery and direct repair.
D. Iliac-brachial veno-venous bypass and repair.
E. Balloon occlusion and removal at 72 hours.

DISCUSSION: The issue with this question is how best to approach a right-sided iliac vein injury or bleeding from the bifurcation of the vena cava when its surgical access is essentially obstructed by the overlying iliac artery and aortic bifurcation. This is best approached by recognizing this dilemma and making a decision to transect the iliac artery. This is then used as a way to mobilize the iliac artery off of the area. Following repair of the vein or vena caval bifurcation, re-anastomosis of the iliac artery into its normal anatomic position is accomplished.

Textbook: Pages 1409–1413 ANSWER: C

9. A 36-year-old man fell from his motorcycle and presents with a supracondylar femur fracture, Grade I tibia fracture, and diminished pulses. The best management would be to:

A. Immediately measure compartment pressures.
B. Start heparin.
C. Begin mannitol diuresis.
D. Go immediately to angiography.
E. Measure the ankle brachial index.

DISCUSSION: This patient presents with a supracondylar femur fracture and diminished pulses. The most important issue is to recognize the critical potential for popliteal artery injury. Failure to recognize arterial injury can lead to popliteal artery thrombosis, and if the thrombosis is not treated in a timely fashion, is almost universally accompanied by amputation. Any patient with posterior knee dislocation, suspicion of knee instability on physical examination, or fractures around the knee joint should raise this diagnosis. Any question about injury should be evaluated with an angiogram.

Textbook: Pages 1413–1416 ANSWER: D

10. A 35-year-old man is ejected from his motorcycle and sustains bilateral femur fractures. Blood pressure is 112/80 and chest x-ray is negative. Computed tomography (CT) scan of the abdomen reveals no significant bleeding. The most reliable indicator of compensated shock is:

A. Orthostatic change in blood pressure.
B. Decreased capillary refill.
C. Urine output less than -50 ml/h.
D. Base excess greater than -5.
E. Cool lower extremities.

DISCUSSION: Shock can occur despite having normal vital signs. It is often overlooked when there is not clear cavitary hemorrhage into the chest or abdomen. The presence of injuries such as bilateral femur fractures is sufficient to lead to compensated shock. The detection of compensated shock requires evaluation for the presence of a lactic acidosis indicating a switch from aerobic to anaerobic metabolism. The base deficit as a surrogate for serum lactate is linearly correlated with mortality. It is a good surrogate and an excellent substitute for serum lactate and is more clinically available than lactate. The routine use of base deficit is wise for assessing patients with multiple injuries in which the presence of compensated shock may not be obvious. Interpretation of the base deficit is generally attributable to hypoperfusion when it is greater than −5. Exceptions would include patients with cocaine metabolites or an individual after a seizure. With these two exceptions, a base deficit greater than −5 is generally a reflection of compensated shock and should improve with appropriate volume resuscitation.

Textbook: Pages 60–63 ANSWER: D

11. A 22-year-old man presents following a motor vehicle crash unconscious and withdrawing the upper and lower extremities to pain. The patient was intubated in the field and arrives normotensive. The most important aspect of initial care to avoid secondary brain injury is:

A. Hyperventilate to a $PaCO_2$ of 25.
B. Intravenous steroids.
C. Sedation with barbiturates.
D. Avoiding hypoxia.
E. Paralysis.

DISCUSSION: This case represents a patient who presents with a severe closed head injury. The potential for secondary injury becomes the focus of initial management, in addition to the diagnosis of a potential space-occupying lesion. The two most important components to avoid in preventing secondary injury include hypotension and hypoxia. In this patient blood pressure is essentially normal and the most important other consideration is the avoidance of hypoxia. Both hypoxia and hypotension and the frequency with which these events occur in the postinjury period are the biggest determinants of outcome for head-injured patients. Recent evidence suggests that hyperventilation below 30 to 35 $PaCO_2$ is contraindicated in head-injured patients and steroids have never been shown to have any benefit.

Textbook: Pages 317–318 ANSWER: D

12. A 22-year-old man was involved in a high-speed motor vehicle crash. On arrival in the trauma suite he is awake and following commands, breathing at a rate of 18 with good bilateral breath sounds. Pulse is 145 and blood pressure is 85/50. The most important priority in resuscitation is:

A. Endotracheal intubation.
B. Identify and control sources of ongoing hemorrhage.
C. Perform bilateral needle thoracostomy.
D. Obtain a complete medical history.
E. Obtain computed tomography (CT) scan of the head.

DISCUSSION: This patient presents with significant trauma and on presentation he is awake and following commands, but hypotensive and tachycardic. Following the primary survey of initial trauma resuscitation he has evidence of an adequate airway. He is breathing and able to follow commands and his breathing is reportedly normal. The next most important priority, particularly in a patient who is awake and following commands, is to re-establish circulation. The components of circulation require the initiation of volume resuscitation and at the same time the quantification of hemorrhage and identification of the source. A relative quantification of hemorrhage can occur from vital signs. A patient who is hypoxic and hypotensive would be assumed to have a Class 3 hemorrhage, or at least a 30% blood volume hemorrhage. The sources for consideration would be obvious lacerations or obvious fractures, and this will account for hypotension approximately 50 to 60% of the time. Cavitary hemorrhage into the chest or abdomen and retroperitoneal hemorrhage due to a pelvic fracture or other retroperitoneal source should be considered as well. A chest x-ray to evaluate cavitary hemorrhage in the chest and an objective evaluation of the abdomen (ultrasound, diagnostic peritoneal lavage, or CT), in addition to obvious evaluation for fractures and lacerations, should be completed quickly. In addition, a pelvic x-ray to suggest a pelvic fracture as a source of hemorrhage should be done.

Textbook: Pages 315–317 ANSWER: B

13. A 34-year-old female has sustained a closed head injury. Computed tomography (CT) of the head is consistent with severe diffuse axonal injury. There are no extra-axial mass lesions. The most important goal of therapy for her head injury is:

A. Osmotic diuresis to achieve serum hyperosmolality.
B. Repair of primary brain injury.
C. Prevention of secondary brain injury.
D. Administration of steroids within the first 24 hours.
E. Establishment of a hyperdynamic state to prevent vasospasm.

DISCUSSION: In this patient with a severe closed head injury, there is no evidence of a space-occupying lesion requiring surgical decompression. The most important management principle for a closed head injury, after making a decision about the need for operation, is the importance of avoiding secondary brain injury. This would include avoiding hypoxia, hypotension, and anything that would contribute to these secondary insults. Excessive hyperventilation, inappropriate elevation of the blood pressure, and failure to adequately resuscitate the patient can all have secondary injury effects. The effects of secondary injury lead to brain swelling and elevation of intracranial pressure and enhance the risk of herniation. The management priorities of everyone caring for the head-injured patient, after the need for operation is established, are aligned around the central focus of avoiding secondary brain injury.

Textbook: Pages 315–317 ANSWER: C

14. A 25-year-old man is involved in a motor vehicle crash. He has an immediate loss of consciousness, and initial Glasgow Coma Scale score of 7. Endotracheal intubation is performed in the field, after neuromuscular blockade. On arrival, the patient is not moving, and he has clear bilateral breath sounds with assisted ventilation. Pulse is 85 and blood pressure is 75 systolic. The best approach is:

A. Resuscitative thoracotomy.
B. Administration of phenylephrine.
C. Administration of isoproterenol.
D. Application of military antishock trousers (MAST).
E. Crystalloid resuscitation and evaluation to identify possible cavitary hemorrhage.

DISCUSSION: This patient presents with a decreased level of consciousness, and is paralyzed and intubated with unclear information about his motor response. His blood pressure is low, but in this case his pulse is also low, suggesting that the normal tachycardic response may not be present. This would occur following a high spinal cord injury, which could also be consistent with a patient who had limited movement and was hypotensive. Although this is a possibility, it is not the initial priority. Hypotension due to bleeding cannot be excluded as the cause of this patient's hypotension until objective evaluation for sources of hemorrhage has been carried out. The use of vasopressors or adjuncts to support cardiac output or blood pressure would be inappropriate until the patient was volume resuscitated and had evaluation for potential sources of hemorrhage completed.

Textbook: Pages 315–317 ANSWER: E

15. A 44-year-old female suffers a single stab wound to the anterior left neck, at approximately the level of the cricoid. There is a visible hematoma, and the patient complains of pain with swallowing. The most appropriate course of action would be:

A. Angiography.
B. Computed tomography (CT) of the neck.
C. Esophagoscopy.
D. Esophagography.
E. Exploration of the neck.

DISCUSSION: The decision to operate on patients with penetrating neck trauma depends on the location of the injury and the initial presentation of symptoms. In a patient who presents with a Zone I or Zone III injury, the use of angiography and other adjunctive diagnostic tests such as esophagography and laryngoscopy will help determine if there is an injury and help plan surgical exposure should surgery be required. The difficulty in surgical exposure for Zone I and Zone III injuries makes routine exploration impractical. Recently, for Zone II injuries, nonoperative evaluation with angiography and esophagography, esophagoscopy, and bronchoscopy has been advocated for wounds of low risk. In this case, the presence of a visible hematoma and pain with swallowing suggest both a significant vascular injury and a significant enteric injury. As such, management would be best with surgery. None of the other options provide for the complete evaluation of all of the potential injuries in the neck and therefore are excluded.

Textbook: Pages 321–324 ANSWER: E

16. Early operative fixation of facial fractures is most likely to be indicated because of:

A. Functional impairment.
B. Cosmetic deformity.
C. Presence of severe multisystem injuries.
D. Loss of teeth.
E. Presence of blood in the maxillary sinus.

DISCUSSION: The early fixation of facial fractures is something that virtually always can be dealt with after more severe injuries have been treated. Loss of teeth, the presence of blood, and even cosmetic deformities can be adequately, and perhaps many times better, treated in a more delayed fashion. The exception to this is when functional impairment to the airway following loss of integrity of the mandible makes early operative fixation essential early in the course of the patient. The decision to do this depends on the initial assessment in detecting functional impairment in this circumstance.

Textbook: Pages 324–326 ANSWER: A

17. What percentage of patients with thoracic trauma require thoracotomy?

A. 10 to 15%.
B. 20 to 25%.
C. 30 to 40%.
D. 45 to 50%.

DISCUSSION: Although chest trauma and hemothorax are very common, the need for thoracotomy is relatively uncommon. The low pressure system in the pulmonary artery and vein makes hemostasis more likely, particularly when the lung is re-expanded and positive-pressure ventilation allows for tamponade. In the presence of a hemothorax, the placement of a chest tube during initial evaluation and ongoing monitoring of blood allow the decision to perform thoracotomy to be made. The goal is complete evacuation and re-expansion of the lung. When there is ongoing hemorrhage, it is usually due to an arterial injury to a subcostal artery or the internal mammary artery or to a significant laceration to the lung. Generally, the initial presentation of greater than 1000 ml blood loss or ongoing hemorrhage of greater than 200 ml/hr becomes an indication for thoracotomy.

Textbook: Pages 326–327 ANSWER: A

18. All of the following radiographic findings indicate a torn thoracic aorta except:

A. Widened mediastinum.
B. Presence of an apical "pleural cap."
C. First rib fractures.
D. Tracheal deviation to the right.
E. Left pneumothorax.

DISCUSSION: The initial evaluation of the patient following a frontal or lateral deceleration mechanism for a torn thoracic aorta is guided by knowledge of the mechanism and initial evaluation of the chest x-ray. Several classic findings on chest x-ray that indicate high suspicion for aortic transection include mediastinal widening, the presence of an apical cap, the association with a first rib fracture, and depression of the tracheal bifurcation with displacement of the trachea to the right and the left mainstem bronchus inferiorly by the hematoma. The presence of a left hemothorax may indicate bleeding and has been reported to be associated with a patient at high risk for early rupture. The presence of a pneumothorax on the left or right has no known association with thoracic aortic injury.

Textbook: Pages 326–331; 1406–1409 ANSWER: E

19. A 28-year-old man was injured in a motorcycle accident in which he was not wearing a helmet. On admission to the emergency room he was in severe respiratory distress and hypotensive (blood pressure 80/40 mm Hg), and appeared cyanotic. He was bleeding profusely from the nose and had an obviously open femur fracture with exposed bone. Breath sounds were decreased on the right side of the chest. The initial management priority should be:

A. Control of hemorrhage with anterior and posterior nasal packing.
B. Tube thoracostomy in the right hemithorax.
C. Endotracheal intubation with in-line cervical traction.
D. Obtain intravenous access and begin emergency type O blood transfusions.
E. Obtain a cross-table cervical spine film and chest film.

DISCUSSION: In this patient there is evidence of respiratory distress and cyanosis and hypotension. The patient is also actively bleeding from his nose and has evidence of increased breath sounds. Given his respiratory distress and cyanosis, the single most important priority becomes establishment of the airway and adequate breathing. Nothing else should be pursued until these priorities are accomplished. Control of hemorrhage, placement of a chest tube, intravenous access, and resuscitation all are important, but until the airway has been established and breathing has commenced, they should not be a focus. The determination of a cervical spine film prior to the placement of an airway when a patient is in respiratory distress is inappropriate, whereas maintaining in-line traction and orotracheal intubation are both safe and lifesaving.

Textbook: Pages 315–317 ANSWER: C

20. Oxygen content of the blood is affected most by:

A. Cardiac output.
B. Hemoglobin concentration.
C. Partial pressure of CO_2.
D. Partial pressure of O_2.

DISCUSSION: Although oxygen delivery is determined by both cardiac output and oxygen content, oxygen content is determined by the equation:

$$O_2 = (1.37 \cdot \%FaO_2 \cdot Hgb) + (0.003 \times PaO_2).$$

Textbook: Page 394 ANSWER: B

21. Common causes of hypoxia in the postoperative surgical patient include all except:

A. Atelectasis.
B. Diffusion defect.
C. Lobar pneumonia.
D. Pulmonary edema.

DISCUSSION: Diffusion defects are an uncommon cause of respiratory failure.

Textbook: Pages 205–208; 394–400 ANSWER: B

22. Impaired mechanics of breathing can occur in all of the following settings except:

A. Phrenic nerve injury.
B. Hypokalemia.
C. Hyperphosphatemia.
D. Guillain-Barré syndrome.

DISCUSSION: Hypophosphatemia, not hyperphosphatemia, can be a cause of impaired ventilatory mechanics.

Textbook: Pages 394–397 ANSWER: C

23. One of the mechanical disadvantages to ventilation associated with the high lung volumes of chronic obstructive pulmonary disease (COPD) is:

A. High intrinsic PEEP.
B. Alveolar flooding.
C. Tracheomalacia.
D. A rounded diaphragm.

DISCUSSION: Air trapping from dynamic airway collapse during exhalation results in high auto PEEP, which is the hallmark of COPD and is partially responsible for the flattened diaphragms of COPD patients.

Textbook: Pages 397–398 ANSWER: A

24. Vital capacity is the lung volume:

A. That remains after forced exhalation.
B. Below which airway collapse begins.
C. The minimum volume to sustain adequate oxygenation and ventilation.
D. Describing the volume of maximal exhalation following a maximal inspiration.

DISCUSSION: Answer A describes residual volumes. Answer B describes closing volume, and Answer C is a deliberate misrepresentation of functional residual capacity.

Textbook: Pages 394–396 ANSWER: D

25. Lung closing volume is:

A. Generally equal to 90% functional residual capacity (FRC).

B. Decreased with smoking.
C. Increased with age of the patient.
D. Rarely seen in postoperative surgical patients.

DISCUSSION: Lung closing volume increases with increasing age and smoking, which, when coupled with reduced FRC in surgical patients, predisposes to airway collapse.

Textbook: Pages 394–397 ANSWER: C

26. First line therapy for bronchospasm is:

A. Nebulized racemic epinephrine.
B. Heliox (40% O_2, 60% helium).
C. Intravenous theophylline.
D. Nebulized beta-agonists

DISCUSSION: Although all of these agents have some efficacy in treating bronchospasm, the first line of treatment should be a nebulized beta-agonist.

Textbook: Page 397 ANSWER: D

27. The following statements regarding the institution of oxygen therapy in patients with chronic obstructive pulmonary disease are all true except:

A. It significantly depresses the drive to breathe.
B. It can be life-sustaining.
C. It may reduce pulmonary artery pressures.
D. It can increase PCO_2.

DISCUSSION: Like any therapeutic intervention, the institution of oxygen therapy should be monitored and titrated to effect. Oxygen has many beneficial effects and does not significantly decrease the drive to breathe.

Textbook: Pages 397–398 ANSWER: A

28. All of the following statements regarding PEEP are true except:

A. If used prophylactically, it can reduce the incidence of adult respiratory distress syndrome.
B. It can recruit functional residual capacity by opening collapsed airways.
C. It can make interpretation of pulmonary artery catheter pressures difficult.
D. At high levels, it can create areas of high $\dot{V}/\dot{Q}$.

DISCUSSION: PEEP can recruit air spaces, raise intrathoracic pressure, and, at high levels, create areas of Zone 1 lung. It cannot prevent ARDS, although it does allow for the reduction of FIO_2.

Textbook: Pages 397–399 ANSWER: A

29. Barotrauma:

A. Rarely occurs with plateau airway pressures less than 50 cm H_2O.
B. Decreases hospital mortality.
C. Is preferable to hypercapnia and respiratory acidosis.
D. Is probably an effect of alveolar overdistention and injury.

DISCUSSION: To reduce barotrauma, plateau pressures should be kept to less than 35 to 40 cm H_2O, and hypercapnia and respiratory acidosis should be tolerated. These strategies have been shown to improve outcomes.

Textbook: Pages 398–399 ANSWER: D

30. The zone of stasis in a burn wound is associated with which of the following?

A. Direct thermal damage.
B. Vasodilation.
C. Neutrophil adherence.
D. Platelet degranulation.
E. Nonnutrient shunting.

DISCUSSION: The zone of stasis is the area immediately adjacent to the irreversibly damaged zone of necrosis caused by direct thermal damage. The zone of stasis is the area that is at risk for further tissue loss due to a relatively low flow state and the localized active destructive inflammatory response associated with neutrophil adherence. Vasodilation and nonnutrient shunting are associated with relatively high blood flows in the zone of hyperemia, which has been associated with platelet degranulation.

Textbook: Page 346 ANSWER: C

31. Deep second-degree wounds re-epithelialize from retained keratinocytes in:

A. Rete ridges.
B. Hair follicles.
C. Moll glands.
D. Reticular dermis.
E. Meissner corpuscles.

DISCUSSION: Deep second-degree burns are defined by the loss of the epidermis, which then re-establishes itself by keratinocyte proliferation from retained epidermal elements in dermal structures, such as hair follicles. The other structures listed are either destroyed or do not contain epidermal elements.

Textbook: Page 346 ANSWER: B

32. A patient with burns to the entire back, scalp (50% of the head and neck), and the posterior thighs has what percentage of his or her total body surface area burned?

A. 40%.
B. 28%.
C. 20%.
D. 32%.
E. 36%.

DISCUSSION: Following the rule of nines, the back is estimated to encompass 18% of the total body surface area (TBSA). The scalp makes up one half of the head and neck, which constitutes 9% of the TBSA. Thus the scalp would contribute 4% to the estimate. Each leg makes up 18% of the TBSA, and the posterior thigh is a little less than one third of the leg. So, adding 18%, 4%, and 10% (2 × 5%) gives a percentage TBSA burned value of 32.

Textbook: Page 347 ANSWER: D

33. Which of the following has been shown to reduce burn wound edema?

A. Methysergide.
B. Aspirin.
C. Diphenhydramine.
D. Nitroprusside.
E. Heparin.

DISCUSSION: Of the above-mentioned compounds, the only substance that has been shown to reduce burn wound edema is methysergide, which is a serotonin antagonist.

Textbook: Pages 347–348 ANSWER: A

34. Severe burns are associated with which of the following immune deficiencies in the acute phase?

A. Neutropenia.
B. Granulocyte colony-stimulating factor deficiency.
C. Polarization to the T-helper 2 (Th2) cell response.
D. Altered macrophage activity.
E. Antibody overproduction.

DISCUSSION: A number of immunologic abnormalities occur in severely burned patients during the initial treatment phase, all leading to immunologic compromise. Among these is a polarization of the dominant T-helper cell phenotype to the relatively immunosuppressive Th2 type. Neutropenia after burns is not common. Granulocyte colony-stimulating factor is actually increased after burn, but the response of the marrow is diminished, leading to decreased macrophage production. Those macrophages that are present remain active.

Textbook: Page 349 ANSWER: C

35. Hypermetabolism in severe burns is related to:

A. Hypocortisolemia.
B. Hepatic glycogen synthesis.
C. Glutamine synthesis.
D. Decreased catecholamine activity.
E. Hyperinsulinemia.

DISCUSSION: Severe burn is perhaps the most potent stimulus for hypermetabolism. This response is associated with increased cortisol and catecholamine levels, increased glucose production by the liver from glycogen stores, and transamination of glucogenic amino acids such as glutamine transported to the liver from the periphery. Insulin levels are actually increased but are relatively ineffective because of insulin resistance.

Textbook: Page 349 ANSWER: E

36. A 40-year-old 100-kg man is involved in a house fire with burns to 45% of his total body surface area (TBSA). He comes to the emergency room with two peripheral intravenous lines which are not being used. It is 2 hours since his injury, and he has not received any resuscitation. His initial intravenous fluid rate should be:

A. 250 ml/hr
B. 500 ml/hr
C. 1000 ml/hr
D. 1500 ml/hr
E. 2000 ml/hr

DISCUSSION: The Parkland formula suggests that the resuscitation volume after severe burn should be 4 ml/kg/% TBSA burned for the first 24 hours after burn, with half given in the first 8 hours and the rest given in the following 16 hours. The formula predicts that this man will require 18,000 ml of isotonic fluid in the first 24 hours after injury (4 × 100 × 45). One half should be given in the first 8 hours after injury. Because resuscitation was not given for 2 hours, 9000 ml should be given over a 6-hour period; thus the initial rate should be 1500 ml/hr.

Textbook: Pages 350–351 ANSWER: D

37. Fasciotomy is indicated in snake venom poisoning:

A. Only when a rattlesnake inflicted the bite.
B. Whenever any pit viper inflicted the bite.
C. Only when there is documented elevation of intracompartmental pressures despite antivenom therapy.
D. Whenever the victim demonstrates a swollen, ecchymotic, painful extremity.

DISCUSSION: Although many patients bitten by pit vipers have very swollen, painful, and discolored extremities, the actual incidence of compartment syndrome is quite low. Most of the venom in these bites is deposited subcutaneously, not intramuscularly. A fasciotomy should be reserved for the rare patient with documented elevations in intracompartmental pressures despite antivenom therapy and elevation of the extremity.

Textbook: Page 366 ANSWER: C

38. Bites by which of the following animals are MOST likely to require rabies prophylaxis?

A. Raccoon.
B. Coral snake.
C. Rabbit.
D. Deer mouse.
E. None of the above.

DISCUSSION: Most rodents (including mice), lagomorphs (rabbits), and all reptiles are not known to transmit rabies. Raccoons, on the other hand, may well carry and transmit the disease. A bite by a wild raccoon that cannot be tested for the presence of the disease should prompt initiation of prophylaxis. If the treating physician is unsure as to whether or not prophylaxis is indicated, a call to the local Public Health Department can be helpful.

Textbook: Pages 367–368 ANSWER: A

39. Commercial antivenoms currently are available in the United States for all of the following animals except:

A. Coral snakes (*Micrurus* species).
B. Widow spiders (*Latrodectus* species).
C. Brown spiders (*Loxosceles* species).
D. Stonefish.

DISCUSSION: There is currently no commercially available antivenom for brown spiders, such as the brown recluse (*Loxosceles reclusa*). Antivenoms are produced in the United States for coral snakes of the genus *Micrurus* and for widow spiders (*Latrodectus* species). Antivenom is produced in Australia for the stonefish. This antivenom is usually available in the United States by contacting regional poison control centers or major marine aquariums.

Textbook: Pages 366, 368, 369, 373 ANSWER: C

40. Which of the following patients is MOST likely to benefit from referral to an allergist for skin testing and possible immunotherapy following a *Hymenoptera* sting?

A. A 6-year-old girl who demonstrates diffuse hives (but no other systemic findings) following a fire ant sting.
B. A 30-year-old man who presents with redness, discomfort, and swelling of his entire right hand and forearm 24 hours following a honeybee sting to his right index finger.
C. A 24-year-old woman who presents with wheezing, diffuse hives, and a blood pressure of 80/40 thirty minutes following a yellow jacket sting.
D. All of the above patients should be referred to an allergist for follow-up.

DISCUSSION: All patients experiencing anaphylaxis following a *Hymenoptera* sting should be referred to an allergist for skin testing and possible desensitization. Children, however, who experience only a dermal response (i.e., diffuse hives) appear to be at no greater risk for a later, more severe reaction, and do not require referral in this setting. Patients who have an exaggerated local reaction (e.g., delayed, severe swelling of the stung extremity) likewise do not require allergy evaluation.

Textbook: Pages 370–371 ANSWER: C

41. Which of the following management principles is NOT appropriate for treating stingray injuries?

A. Immersing the injured extremity in hot, nonscalding water.
B. Obtaining radiographs of the extremity.
C. Routinely exploring the local wound.
D. Performing prompt, primary closure.

DISCUSSION: Immersing the painful, stung extremity in hot, nonscalding water serves to deactivate the heat-labile toxins at work. Radiographs may identify pieces of spine left in the wound. The site should be routinely explored and irrigated under appropriate local/regional anesthesia to assess for foreign bodies and to débride/cleanse the wound. Primary closure should be avoided, as this greatly increases the risk of secondary infection. Instead, the wound should be allowed to heal by secondary intention or should be closed in a delayed fashion.

Textbook: Page 373 ANSWER: D

42. A multiple-injury trauma patient, who is septic 10 days after injury, has become oliguric and has a decreased creatinine clearance. Which of the following should be initiated as therapy for his renal failure?

A. A continuous dopamine infusion 3 μg/kg/min.
B. Reduce protein intake by changing the enteral feeding formula.
C. Intermittent hemodialysis every other day.
D. Continuous renal replacement therapy (e.g., complete venovenous hemodiafiltration [CVVHD]).
E. A continuous furosemide infusion.

DISCUSSION: The use of pharmacologic therapy in acute renal failure in critically ill patients has not been shown to be of benefit. An example of the lack of evidence is cited. The advantage of CVVHD over intermittent hemodialysis (IHD) is superior hemodynamic stability, particularly in patients with the potential for occult regional hypoperfusion. Theoretical advantage and expert opinion (Society of Critical Care Medicine [SCCM] meeting) support this; no Class 3 or Class 4 evidence exists. Finally, no evidence exists that withholding protein improves outcome, as this is a strategy for chronic renal failure patients.

Textbook: Page 386 ANSWER: D

43. Colloid solutions are preferred over crystalloid solutions in resuscitation from hemorrhagic shock for the following reason:

A. Improved oxygenation due to less lung water.
B. Colloids demonstrate no benefit over crystalloids.
C. Maintaining oncotic pressure decreases multiple organ failure.
D. Less renal failure.
E. Better survival.

DISCUSSION: There is no evidence to date that colloid administration improved outcome in critically ill patients, or the subgroups of trauma patients.

Textbook: Pages 380–381 ANSWER: B

44. Which of the following should be instituted as the primary therapy in the care of a patient with a severe closed-head injury and intracranial pressure greater than 25?

A. Diuretics (e.g., mannitol) to reduce cerebral edema.
B. Hyperventilation ($PaCO_2$ <30 mm Hg).
C. Barbiturate coma.

D. Intravenous methylprednisolone (Solu-Medrol) to reduce cerebral edema.
E. Intravenous hydration to restore euvolemia and maintain cerebral perfusion pressure (CPP).

DISCUSSION: Recent studies suggest the re-establishment of global cerebral perfusion (measured via CPP) as the number one priority in the treatment of cerebral trauma. This comes from a number of studies examining improved blood flow in cerebral injury.
Textbook: Pages 375–376 ANSWER: E

45. The most common cause of right ventricular failure among surgical patients is:
A. Cardiac contusion from blunt trauma.
B. Primary pulmonary hypertension.
C. Right heart myocardial ischemia from coronary artery disease.
D. Pulmonary hypertension secondary to the adult respiratory distress syndrome (ARDS).
E. Pulmonary valve stenosis.

DISCUSSION: As discussed in the excellent review paper by Calvin (1991), the most common cause of right heart failure is due to increased pulmonary vascular resistance from pulmonary pathology (secondary right heart failure). In surgical patients the most common cause is acute lung injury and ARDS from a myriad of causes. Primary pulmonary hypertension and primary right ventricular pathologies are extremely rare.
Textbook: Page 379 ANSWER: D

46. Which of the following is not a symptom of adrenal insufficiency among surgical patients with prolonged intensive care unit stay?
A. Persistent hypokalemia.
B. Failure of catecholamine administration to raise mean arterial pressure.
C. Eosinophilia.
D. Unexplained hypoglycemia.
E. Hypotension despite adequate vascular volume (euvolemia).

DISCUSSION: Adrenal insufficiency results in all of the above except hypokalemia (hyperkalemia is the usual manifestation).
Textbook: Page 388 ANSWER: A

47. Administration of which vasocative medication usually improves gastric mucosal (pH_i) CO_2 concentration along with its other beneficial effects?
A. Dopamine.
B. Epinephrine.
C. Dobutamine.
D. Phenylephrine.
E. Norepinephrine.

DISCUSSION: Intestinal regional hypoperfusion is associated with multiple organ failure and decreased survival. The effects of multiple catecholamines are unpredictable, but in general all of those listed except for dobutamine have some beneficial effects.
Textbook: Pages 63–65; 380–381 ANSWER: C

48. Which of the following is least likely to occur in a trauma patient with a poorly controlled retroperitoneal hemorrhage from a complex pelvic fracture, who now has developed a measured bladder pressure of 32 mm Hg?
A. An increasing intracranial pressure.
B. An elevated mean airway pressure.
C. Anuria.
D. Falling cardiac output due to lower stroke volume.
E. Reflex bradycardia causing hypotension.

DISCUSSION: The manifestations and pathophysiology of abdominal compartment syndrome include decreased cardiac output, renal failure, respiratory failure, intracranial hypertension, and internal and hepatic ischemia (Saggi et al., 1998). No reflex bradycardia has been described.
Textbook: Page 382 ANSWER: E

49. Which of the following is not an indication to initiate stress gastritis prophylaxis on an intensive care unit patient?
A. Respiratory failure requiring mechanical ventilation.
B. Proximal enterocutaneous fistula with the patient on total parenteral nutrition (TPN).
C. A history of gastrointestinal bleeding.
D. Severe cerebral injury.
E. Coagulopathy.

DISCUSSION: A large body of literature exists (mostly Class 2 and Class 3 data) defining the indications for stress ulcer prophylaxis. TPN, administered for whatever reason, has not been found to require stress ulcer prophylaxis.
Textbook: Page 381 ANSWER: B

50. Which of the following statements concerning early enteral nutrition is false?
A. When compared to total parenteral nutrition (TPN), enteral nutrition (EN) is associated with less septic morbidity.
B. Eighty-five percent of intensive care unit patients will reach their nutritional goals in 5 days.
C. EN prevents intestinal mucosal atrophy.
D. EN maintains normal intestinal flora.
E. If EN is not tolerated in the first 48 hours, TPN should be initiated.

DISCUSSION: There are no data to support short-term (<7 days) use of TPN in patients who previously were not malnourished (McQuiggan et al., 1999).
Textbook: Pages 101–117; 387–388 ANSWER: E

51. Which of the following concerning thyroid function in critically ill patients is false?
A. Triiodothyronine (T_3) and thyroxin (T_4) binding protein concentrations decrease.

B. Dopamine administration may decrease thyroid-stimulating hormone (TSH) levels.
C. The *sick euthyroid state* (i.e., low T_3 and T_4, high resin T_3, and normal free T_4 and TSH) should be aggressively treated with thyroid hormone replacement.
D. Cortisol secretion may decrease TSH levels.
E. Elevated TSH levels are not expected and may suggest functional hypothyroidism.

DISCUSSION: The sick euthyroid state is not well understood, and no data exist that indicate replacement therapy improves outcome.

Textbook: Page 388 ANSWER: C

52. Which of the following concerning the coagulopathy after massive transfusion is false?

A. Coagulation factor depletion is associated with hypothermia and metabolic acidosis.
B. Factor replacement of 6 units of platelets and 2 units of fresh frozen plasma for every 10 units of packed red blood cells has been shown to be effective therapy.
C. Complications of massive transfusion include hyperkalemia, hypocalcemia, and hypomagnesemia.
D. Mechanical control of large vessel hemorrhage is the highest priority.
E. Factor replacement should be guided by clinical signs of bleeding, laboratory abnormalities, and point of care testing.

DISCUSSION: No Class 1 or Class 2 data exist supporting a "formula" approach to factor replacement. There are data to support the concept that early surgical control reduces the magnitude of the subsequent coagulopathy. Since no data exist to the contrary, a conservative strategy that limits the use of blood products is recommended by most experts.

Textbook: Pages 389–390 ANSWER: B

53. Treatment of a postoperative surgical patient with a mean arterial pressure (MAP) of 60 mm Hg, an arterial pH of 7.28, and suspected left heart failure should include:

A. Diuresis with furosemide to correct fluid overload.
B. Esmolol drip to reduce myocardial oxygen demand.
C. Intravenous fluid bolus followed by echocardiography.
D. Bicarbonate drip to correct the pH.
E. Nitroprusside for afterload reduction.

DISCUSSION: Hypovolemia is a much more common cause of shock in the surgical intensive care unit than left ventricular failure. Aggressive diuresis when the cause of shock has not been confirmed can add to the problem, and would likely be ineffective with a MAP of 60 mm Hg (poor renal perfusion). Beta-blockade can also compound the problem if the patient is relatively hypovolemic by preventing an increased heart rate from supporting a low stroke volume. No data exist demonstrating an improved outcome with acid buffering in the uncorrected shock state. Afterload reduction would be extremely dangerous in a patient with a MAP of 60 mm Hg, tending to reduce it further. The correct strategy is a moderate fluid bolus to improve preload, because the left ventricle becomes less compliant in most cases and develops diastolic dysfunction. Increased preload improves diastolic filling and, thus, stroke volume. This is a temporizing measure until a more definite characterization of the cardiac dysfunction can be done with echocardiography or invasive monitoring.

Textbook: Pages 377–381 ANSWER: C

54. The signs and symptoms of cardiac tamponade include all of the following except:

A. Pulsus paradoxus (decreased systolic blood pressure >10 mm Hg with inspiration).
B. Distended neck veins.
C. Decreased mean arterial pressure.
D. Decreased amplitude of the QRS complex on electrocardiography.
E. Accentuated S_2 heart sound.

DISCUSSION: These are classic descriptors of the clinical diagnosis of cardiac tamponade. So-called muffled heart sounds are classically described, not the accentuated S_2 in the question. This question is included because tamponade can occur for a variety of reasons in the surgical intensive care unit, has an insidious onset, and must be recognized by clinical examination to be corrected.

Textbook: Pages 379–380 ANSWER: E

NOTES

NOTES

NOTES

CHAPTER 6

TRANSPLANTATION

1. Which of the following is NOT a correct pairing of immunosuppressive drug and side effect?

A. Mycophenolate mofetil and leukopenia.
B. Cyclosporine and hypertension.
C. Tacrolimus and nephrotoxicity.
D. Daclizumab and serum sickness.
E. Prednisone and cataract formation.

DISCUSSION: Daclizumab and basiliximab are new immunosuppressive drugs, that prevent rejection by binding to the high-affinity interleukin-2 receptor on activated T cells. These drugs are very well tolerated. Serum sickness is seen with antilymphocyte globulins made from horse or rabbit sera. OKT3 can cause a cytokine release syndrome. The other pairings are correct.

Textbook: Page 422 ANSWER: D

2. Cyclosporine and tacrolimus share as a mechanism of action:

A. Antimetabolites that block purine synthesis.
B. Lymphocyte depletion through opsonization.
C. Inhibition of interleukin-2 (IL-2) production.
D. Blockade of high-affinity IL-2 receptors.
E. Inhibition of signal transduction from IL-2 receptor to nucleus.

DISCUSSION: Cyclosporine and tacrolimus block IL-2 production. Azathioprine and mycophenolate mofteil are antimetabolites. Daclizumab and basiliximab block high-affinity IL-2 receptors. Sirolimus inhibits transduction of signals from the IL-2 receptor to the nucleus.

Textbook: Page 423 ANSWER: C

3. Chronic rejection presents as fibrosis and scarring in organs currently transplanted. Probable cause(s) of chronic rejection is (are):

A. Donor factors such as hypertension and age.
B. Preformed antibodies against donor tissue.
C. Previous acute rejection episodes.
D. A and C.
E. All of the above.

DISCUSSION: Chronic rejection is poorly understood, but currently is believed to be caused by immunologic factors as well as other donor and recipient factors. Risk factors for development of chronic rejection include (1) previous acute rejection episodes; (2) inadequate immunosuppression, including noncompliance; (3) initial delayed graft function; (4) donor issues such as age and hypertension; (5) organ recovery issues; and (6) recipient hypertension, diabetes, or infection. Preformed antibodies cause hyperacute rejection.

Textbook: Page 415 ANSWER: D

4. MHC Class II molecules:

A. Are associated with HLA-DR.
B. Interact with $CD8^+$ T cells.
C. Are expressed on almost all cells of an adult.
D. A and C.
E. All of the above.

DISCUSSION: MHC Class I molecules are (1) expressed on most cells; (2) associated with HLA-A and -B; and (3) interact with $CD8^+$ T cells. MHC Class II molecules are (1) expressed only on dendritic cells, B lymphocytes, macrophages, and endothelial cells (after stimulation with cytokines); (2) associated with HLA-DR, -DQ, and -DP; and (3) interact with $CD4^+$ T cells.

Textbook: Page 413 ANSWER: A

5. Acute rejection:

A. Is prevented by screening the recipient for preformed antibodies.
B. Is mediated primarily by T lymphocytes.
C. Always occurs in the first year after transplant.
D. Is not prevented by immunosuppressive drugs.
E. Pathologically presents as allograft fibrosis.

DISCUSSION: Acute rejection is mediated primarily by T lymphocytes. It is most common in the first 3 to 6 months after transplant, but can occur anytime after transplant. Noncompliance with immunosuppressive drugs can contribute to the development of both acute and chronic rejection. Immunosuppressive drugs are designed to prevent acute rejection; screening for preformed antibodies prevents hyperacute rejection only. Acute rejection presents as a lymphocytic infiltrate in the graft. Fibrosis is seen in chronic rejection of all types of organ allografts.

Textbook: Page 424 ANSWER: B

6. The presence of donor-reactive lymphocytotoxic antibodies in the serum of a potential kidney transplant recipient:

A. Can be detected by in vitro testing with recipient leukocytes and donor serum.

B. Is a contraindication to kidney transplantation.
C. Can be found in all male patients more than 20 years of age.

DISCUSSION: The presence of donor-reactive antibodies, detected by incubation of the recipient serum with donor lymphocytes in the presence of complement, results in a "positive crossmatch," and is a contraindication to renal transplantation. The antibodies occur as a result of pregnancy, blood transfusions, or previous organ transplants.

Textbook: Page 431 ANSWER: B

7. Use of a living-related donor instead of a cadaveric donor is no longer an advantage in renal transplantation because:

A. Public recognition of transplantation as a successful therapy has facilitated obtaining family permission for recovery of transplantable organs. Thus, sufficient kidneys from "brain-dead" accident victims are available, obviating the need to use related donors.
B. The results of cadaveric renal transplants under cyclosporine and other modern drug therapy have improved their outcome, which is now as good as that of related donor transplants.
C. Modern preservation techniques can maintain the viability of kidneys from cadaveric donors for many hours, consistently allowing their early function to be as good as that of kidneys from living donors.
D. None of the above.

DISCUSSION: There is general acceptance that transplantation is a useful therapy; however, the number of recipients continues to greatly exceed the number of suitable cadaveric donors whose families grant permission for organ recovery. Thus, availability of a living donor may shorten the waiting period for a transplant by several years. Modern immunosuppression has improved the short-term results of cadaveric transplantation but the attrition of these grafts is greater than living donor transplants, especially those with close histocompatibility. Although preservation techniques can maintain viable kidneys for 36 to 48 hours, cadaveric kidneys suffer a higher rate of posttransplant acute tubular necrosis than those from living donors. Delayed function is adversely associated with long-term function. None of the answers is correct.

Textbook: Page 432 ANSWER: D

8. Survival rates of patients on dialysis are better than those of patients receiving renal allografts in the following circumstances:

A. A living-related donor is available.
B. A cadaver donor must be used.
C. The recipient's renal failure is secondary to diabetes.
D. None of the above.

DISCUSSION: Patients undergoing chronic dialysis have a mortality rate of 6 to 20% per year, every year. This mortality is as high as 11 to 25% per year in diabetic dialysis patients. Patients undergoing renal transplantation have an operative mortality rate of less than 2% and the 1-year survival rate of recipients of living-related donor kidneys is greater than 95%. Survival is greater than 90% for recipients of cadaveric kidneys. Five-year patient survivals are approximately 80% for nondiabetic recipients of living-related and cadaver kidneys, and 60 to 70% for diabetic recipients. Thus, a well-functioning renal allograft provides a greater chance for a longer life than does chronic dialysis. None of the answers is correct.

Textbook: Page 446 ANSWER: D

9. Posttransplantation hypertension can be caused by:

A. Rejection.
B. Cyclosporine nephrotoxicity.
C. Renal transplant artery stenosis (RTAS).
D. Recurrent disease in the allograft.
E. All of the above.

DISCUSSION: Both acute and chronic rejection may result in hypertension. The former causes acute fluid retention and plugging of peritubular capillaries with inflammatory cells. This may progress to intimal swelling and medial necrosis and eventuate in ischemia secondary to endothelial proliferation and obliteration of small vessels. Chronic rejection, thought to be related to protracted humoral injury, results in obliteration of capillaries via the development of intimal hyperplasia. Cyclosporine has a vasoconstrictive effect which, through activation of the renin-angiotensin system, may lead to hypertension. RTAS is responsible for hypertension in 4 to 12% of renal allograft recipients. It responds well to percutaneous angioplasty. A careful trial of angiotensin-converting enzyme inhibitors may be diagnostic of RTAS. Recurrent disease such as membranoproliferative glomerulonephritis and focal glomerular sclerosis may result in significant hypertension in renal allograft recipients. All of the answers are correct.

Textbook: Page 441 ANSWER: E

10. Regarding posttransplantation malignancy, which of the following statements is correct?

A. Certain immunosuppressive agents increase the incidence of malignancy in transplant recipients, while others do not.
B. Those malignancies most commonly seen in the general population (breast, colon) have a substantially greater incidence in transplant recipients.
C. Lymphoproliferative states and B-cell lymphomas are associated with Epstein-Barr virus.

DISCUSSION: Both naturally occurring and iatrogenic states of immune deficiency are associated with an increased rate of de novo malignancy. Transplant recipients have a rate of malignancy approximating 100 times that of the normal population. The degree of immunosuppression rather than a specific immunosuppressive agent appears to be responsible. Squamous and basal cell carcinomas of the skin are most common in the general population. However, other tumors that occur commonly in the general population such as breast and colon cancers do not appear to be increased in incidence. Lymphomas, which occur at a rate that is 350 times normal, and the lymphoproliferative states, which often precede them, appear to be associated with Epstein-Barr virus. Possible explanations of these high malignancy rates include defective immunosurveillance, chronic stimulation of the reticuloendothelial system by the allograft, the carcinogenic effect of immunosuppressive drugs, and viral oncogenesis.

Textbook: Page 444 ANSWER: C

11. Contraindications to liver transplantation include:

A. Fulminant hepatic failure with hepatic coma.
B. Chronic active hepatitis.
C. Hepatic malignancy.
D. Portal vein thrombosis.
E. Uncontrolled sepsis.

DISCUSSION: Fulminant hepatic failure is a common indication for transplantation and the presence of coma is frequent. Unless irreversible neurologic injury has occurred, expeditious transplantation can be lifesaving. Chronic hepatitis with hepatitis B and hepatitis C constitutes the most common indication for transplantation. Hepatocellular malignancy that is confined to the liver is a frequent indication for transplantation, although it is generally limited to single tumors that are less than 6 cm and lack macrovascular infiltration. Recipient portal vein thrombosis was once considered by many to preclude transplantation. With recent technical advances it is now handled routinely with little sequelae in most cases. Uncontrolled sepsis in the recipient is likely to be exacerbated by peritransplant immunosuppression, and is a formal contraindication to transplantation.

Textbook: Page 447 ANSWER: E

12. An abrupt elevation in liver enzymes (transaminases) 1 week after transplant in a previously well functioning adult graft is most likely due to:

A. Cytomegalovirus (CMV) hepatitis.
B. Recurrent hepatitis C.
C. Acute cellular rejection.
D. Anastomotic biliary stricture.
E. Hepatic artery thrombosis.

DISCUSSION: CMV is a common opportunistic infection after transplant but generally occurs later than 1 week postoperatively. Similarly, hepatitis C is likely to reinfect the transplanted liver in a recipient who carries the virus; however, it is more likely to affect liver function at a later time after the transplant. Biliary strictures are generally manifest by elevation in other liver function tests, such as alkaline phosphatase, GGT, and total bilirubin, although mild transaminase elevations can also be evident. Strictures are unlikely at 1 week after transplant. Both hepatic artery thrombosis and acute cellular rejection are potential explanations for enzyme elevations at 1 week after transplant. Hepatic artery thrombosis, however, is quite infrequent, occurring in less than 2% of adult transplants. Acute cellular rejection occurs in up to 30% of liver transplants by 6 months and has a peak onset of 1 to 2 weeks after transplant.

Textbook: Page 452 ANSWER: C

13. Exocrine secretions from a pancreas transplant should be handled by:

A. Placing the transplanted pancreas into the lesser sac and anastomosing the donor duodenal segment to the stomach.
B. Ligating the pancreatic duct.
C. Draining the secretions either into the gastrointestinal or urinary tract by anastomosing the donor duodenal segment to the small bowel or bladder, respectively.
D. Leaving the pancreatic duct open, allowing pancreatic juice to drain freely into the peritoneal cavity, from which it will be reabsorbed.

DISCUSSION: In early experimental pancreas transplants, duct ligation and drainage of exocrine secretions into the peritoneal cavity were employed, sometimes successfully. However, the best clinical results have been obtained with drainage into the bladder or the small intestine. Either of these methods is acceptable, but gastrointestinal drainage is gaining greater acceptance because it avoids the need for bicarbonate replacement and the urethritis that sometimes occurs with bladder drainage.

Textbook: Page 455 ANSWER: C

14. Which of the following is true about transplantation of the small intestine?

A. Clinical graft-versus-host disease occurs in 50% of individuals receiving a small intestinal graft from an allogeneic donor.
B. Patient and graft survival is improved when a liver graft is transplanted simultaneously with a small intestinal graft.
C. The primary cause of death after a small bowel transplant is malnutrition.
D. The primary cause of graft failure is rejection.
E. Posttransplant lymphoproliferative disease is uncommon following small bowel transplantation.

DISCUSSION: Graft-versus-host disease is 5- to 10-fold more common than with solid organ transplants and affects approximately 5% of recipients. This is likely a result of the large mass of immunocompetent donor lymphoid tissue transferred with the graft. Patient

and graft survival are not significantly different in small bowel or small bowel plus liver grafts. Sepsis is by far the most frequent cause of death following small intestinal transplants and is most likely due to the intense immunosuppression required to avoid graft rejection and the loss of the intestinal mucosal barrier in failing grafts. Rejection is the primary barrier to successful small bowel transplantation and is responsible for graft loss in approximately 50% of cases. Posttransplant lymphoproliferative disorder occurs in approximately 10% of small bowel recipients.
Textbook: Page 466 ANSWER: D

NOTES

NOTES

CHAPTER 7

SURGICAL ONCOLOGY

1. Which of the following genetic changes may be involved in tumorigenesis?

A. Activation of a proto-oncogene.
B. Loss of a tumor suppressor gene.
C. Activation of a growth factor receptor–encoding gene.
D. All of the above.

DISCUSSION: Tumors are characterized by uncontrolled cell division. Therefore, genetic changes in genes that control cell division may contribute to tumorigenesis.

Textbook: Page 480 ANSWER: D

2. Do T lymphocytes prevent initiation of non–virally induced tumors?

A. Yes, but sometimes an individual's T cell repertoire has holes.
B. Yes, but sometimes tumor cells escape.
C. No, since early tumor cells may not be antigenic.
D. No, because tumor-bearing patients are immunosuppressed.

DISCUSSION: The incidence of tumors is not increased in T cell–deficient or immunosuppressed individuals, suggesting that T cells do not prevent initiation. Immunosuppression becomes apparent at later stages of tumor development.

Textbook: Page 475 ANSWER: C

3. Which type of treatment, after surgery, may provide the best treatment alternative for eradication of microscopic disease?

A. Chemotherapy.
B. Radiation therapy.
C. Immunotherapy.
D. Combination therapy.

DISCUSSION: Because chemotherapy, radiation therapy, and immunotherapy work through different mechanisms, combination therapy may work the best.

Textbook: Page 477 ANSWER: D

4. Which of the following is currently the most commonly used application of tumor marker evaluation?

A. To aid diagnostics.
B. To determine prognosis.
C. To determine therapeutic strategy.
D. To determine a prophylactic treatment strategy.

DISCUSSION: All tumor markers that are used to determine treatment or prognosis are automatically diagnostic markers but not the other way around.

Textbook: Page 482 ANSWER: A

5. Germline mutations have been postulated to be associated with several tumors. Which of the following is an example?

A. p53.
B. APC.
C. K-*ras*.
D. All of the above.

DISCUSSION: Mutations in the tumor suppressor gene p53 and in the oncogene K-*ras* are acquired mutations, common to many types of tumors. Mutations in the APC gene, however, are germline mutations that may give rise to familial adenomatous polyposis.

Textbook: Page 472 ANSWER: B

6. Factors that limit local recurrence in extremity soft tissue sarcoma include all except:

A. Complete local resection.
B. Histologically negative margins.
C. Adjuvant radiation therapy.
D. Neoadjuvant chemotherapy.
E. Primary presentation.

DISCUSSION: Although neoadjuvant chemotherapy is an approach to the high-risk (large, deep, high-grade) patient, it has not proved to be a factor in decreasing local recurrence.

Textbook: Page 515 ANSWER: D

7. Risk factors for local recurrence in extremity soft tissue sarcoma include all of the following except:

A. Positive microscopic margin.
B. Fibrosarcoma histopathology.
C. Deep location.
D. High histologic grade.
E. Previous recurrence.

DISCUSSION: The predominant risk factors for local recurrence are positive margin and previous local recurrence. Some histopathologic types such as fibrosarcoma have a greater risk for local recurrence than others.

Textbook: Page 517 ANSWER: C

8. Risk factors for distant metastasis in extremity soft tissue sarcoma include all of the following except:

A. Recurrent presentation.
B. Size greater than 10 cm.
C. Deep location.
D. Fibrosarcoma histopathology.
E. High histologic grade.

DISCUSSION: Size, grade, depth, and recurrent presentation are all associated with subsequent risk of metastasis. Fibrosarcomas tend to have a high local recurrence rate, but as a histologic subtype they have a lower risk of metastasis.

Textbook: Page 517 ANSWER: D

9. True statements about soft tissue sarcomas include which of the following?

A. Approximately 50% occur in the extremities.
B. Prior radiation therapy is an etiologic agent.
C. Lymphedema is a predisposing factor.
D. Liposarcoma is the most common histopathology.
E. All of the above.

DISCUSSION: All of these factors are true.

Textbook: Page 512 ANSWER: E

10. Important poor prognostic factors for survival in extremity soft tissue sarcoma include which of the following?

A. High histologic grade.
B. Liposarcoma histopathology.
C. Size less than 8 cm.
D. Distal limb site.
E. Prior incisional biopsy.

DISCUSSION: The major factors for survival in extremity soft tissue sarcoma are the factors that are associated with metastasis. The major factor in the extremity is high histologic grade, although with time large size (>8 cm) assumes greater importance.

Textbook: Page 517 ANSWER: A

11. Which of the following is true of the epidemiology and etiology of melanoma?

A. Most patients are diagnosed after age 60.
B. Skin color has no association with the risk of melanoma.
C. Sun exposure is the only risk factor for melanoma.
D. The highest per capita incidence of melanoma is in Australia.

DISCUSSION: The median age at diagnosis is in the late 40s; therefore a minority of patients are diagnosed after age 60. The risk of melanoma is closely tied to skin color, with Caucasians at highest risk, and those with a Celtic complexion at even higher risk. Australia has a large Celtic population near the equator, and it has the highest per capita incidence of melanoma in the world. Sun exposure is believed to be an important causative factor for melanoma, but those data remain incomplete. There are melanomas that arise in sites not exposed to the sun (e.g., mucous membranes); thus sun exposure is not the only risk factor.

Textbook: Page 487 ANSWER: D

12. Which of the following best predicts the prognosis of patients with a recent diagnosis of cutaneous melanoma and no clinical evidence of metastatic disease?

A. Breslow thickness.
B. Clark level.
C. Ulceration.
D. Gender.
E. Celtic complexion.

DISCUSSION: The prognosis of a patient with melanoma is best predicted by the thickness, measured in millimeters (Breslow thickness). Clark level and ulceration are also predictive, but less so. Gender is a secondary prognostic factor. Skin color may have a mild impact on outcome, but is primarily a risk factor for developing melanoma.

Textbook: Page 494 ANSWER: A

13. A 38-year-old man presents with a melanoma of the skin of the right calf; the tumor is 5 mm thick. Several large nodes are palpable in the R inguinal region. Which of the following is false regarding the appropriate management of this clinical problem?

A. In the absence of systemic disease, the primary melanoma of the right calf should be excised with at least a 2-cm margin.
B. A complete right inguinal node dissection should be performed if there is no evidence of systemic metastasis.
C. If further work-up reveals multiple bilateral lung metastases of melanoma, then they should be excised as soon as possible.
D. Chemotherapy is primarily palliative for melanoma; therefore, surgical therapy is preferred if there is no evidence of metastastic disease beyond the inguinal region.

DISCUSSION: This patient should be evaluated with computed tomography scanning in addition to a careful history, review of systems, and physical examination. If there is no evidence of metastatic disease beyond the inguinal region, then therapy should be focused on the local and regional disease. The primary lesion should be excised with a 2-cm margin. The enlarged nodes can be evaluated by fine-needle aspiration (FNA), or node excision. If the FNA or excisional biopsy does show metastatic melanoma, then a complete inguinal node dissection should be performed. Alternatively, a complete node dissection can be justified simply based on the clinical findings. Chemotherapy does not provide any significant chance of cure, although a significant proportion of patients with isolated nodal metastases live long-term. If work-up does reveal systemic disease, chemotherapy or experimental systemic therapies should be considered. Surgery does not have a therapeutic role in multiple lung metastases of melanoma, although it is occasionally performed as a heroic measure in rare cases. In such cases, however, it is reasonable to observe the patient for a brief period to rule out new metastases prior to any heroic resection of distant disease.

Textbook: Page 455 ANSWER: C

14. The best approach for management of a 2-cm basal cell cancer of the right cheek is:

A. Radical resection with a 2-cm gross margin.
B. Radical resection with radiation therapy.
C. Chemotherapy.
D. Mohs' surgery.
E. Mohs' surgery with radiation therapy.

DISCUSSION: Basal cell cancers almost always grow as a solid contiguous mass, but with extensions into the soft tissue that may be quite long. Resection margins are very well controlled by serial resection and examination of the margins en face (Mohs' surgery), and no adjuvant therapy should be needed in cases with negative margins. Especially on the face, avoidance of radical resection is desirable, and Mohs' surgery provides excellent control of margins with minimal resection.

Textbook: Page 503 ANSWER: D

15. Which of the following is not true about angiosarcoma?

A. Angiosarcomas may occur in the breast many years after radiation therapy.
B. Lymphedema predisposes to angiosarcoma.
C. The most common risk factor for angiosarcoma is sun exposure to superficial blood vessels.
D. Local control of angiosarcomas is difficult to obtain by wide resection and radiation therapy.

DISCUSSION: Angiosarcomas are well described as radiation-induced tumors that occur after radiation therapy for breast cancer, and they are also observed in association with chronic lymphedema. However, sun exposure is not a known risk factor. Unfortunately, local control is very difficult to obtain in most cases.

Textbook: Page 504 ANSWER: C

16. The genetic basis of melanoma is being elucidated in part. A genetic abnormality commonly associated with familial melanoma is also associated with another human cancer. The gene involved, and the associated malignancy, is which of the following?

A. p53, pancreatic cancer.
B. telomerase, retinoblastoma.
C. p16, glioblastoma.
D. p53, glioblastoma.
E. p16, pancreatic cancer.

DISCUSSION: Commonly, mutations in p16 are observed in familial melanoma. These mutations are also found in pancreatic cancer.

Textbook: Page 488 ANSWER: E

17. In a 35-year-old woman with a 1.4-mm-thick melanoma of the right upper thigh, sentinel node biopsy should be offered in which of the following cases?

A. The patient has one child who is 15 years old, and she and her husband are considering having another child but they don't want to proceed if she is at high risk for mortality from the melanoma.
B. The patient wants to be enrolled in an experimental protocol if there is evidence for metastatic disease.
C. There are no contraindications to interferon therapy, and the patient wants to know if she should start interferon therapy.
D. There are several 5- to 8-mm shotty nodes palpable in the right groin.
E. A well-circumscribed 6-mm subcutaneous nodule on the left shoulder is evaluated by fine-needle aspiration and found also to contain melanoma cells.

DISCUSSION: The prognostic information provided the mother who is considering expanding her family is of significant value, and justifies a sentinel node biopsy for staging. Any patient who is a candidate for adjuvant therapy should be offered sentinel node biopsy if the finding of a positive node would make that patient eligible for the therapy. With negative nodes, a patient with a 1.3-mm primary lesion is not a candidate for interferon or for experimental vaccine therapy. The presence of shotty nodes in the nodal basin is not a contraindication to sentinel node biopsy; however, the finding of a node with metastatic melanoma is a contraindication; that patient should undergo therapeutic lymph node dissection. The finding of a distant metastasis, whether in viscera or in the skin, is diagnosed as Stage IV; so the sentinel node biopsy adds nothing to the staging or treatment of the patient with a distant skin metastasis.

Textbook: Page 495 ANSWER: E

18. A 60-year-old woman has a basal cell carcinoma (BCC) of the nose. Her risk of developing another skin cancer elsewhere in the next 5 years is:

A. 0%.
B. 25%.
C. 50%.
D. 75%.
E. 100%.

DISCUSSION: An individual who develops one BCC or squamous cell cancer has an estimated risk of developing one or more additional skin cancers of 35% at 3 years and 50% at 5 years.

Textbook: Page 501 ANSWER: C

19. Squamous cell cancers (SCC) that develop in which one of the following locations have the highest metastatic rate?

A. Hand.
B. Trunk.

C. Nose.
D. Lip.
E. Arm.

DISCUSSION: Anatomic site appears to play an important role in the behavior of SCC. Both the ear and lip are consistently reported to have elevated recurrence and metastatic rates. Other locations that have increased risk for recurrence and metastasis are the nasolabial creases and the periorbital and preauricular regions.
Textbook: Page 501 ANSWER: D

20. The most likely histologic subtype of basal cell carcinoma (BCC) to have clinically undetected tumor extension and require larger surgical margins is:

A. Nodular.
B. Superficial.
C. Infiltrative.
D. Cystic.
E. Pigmented.

DISCUSSION: BCC of any histologic subtype can have malignant extension that is invisible to the eye, but micronodular, infiltrative, and morpheaform are consistently deceptive and actually much larger than they clinically appear to be compared with other histologic subtypes of BCC. Micronodular, infiltrative, and morpheaform BCC often need large excision margins to completely remove tumor.
Textbook: Page 502 ANSWER: C

21. Biopsy of a primary bone tumor should be:

A. Done as soon as the lesion is discovered.
B. Done after thorough staging studies are completed.
C. Done in the operating room.
D. Done at the same time that the venous access port is placed.

DISCUSSION: A careful work-up is required. This may include a full staging evaluation with bone scan, chest computed tomography (CT), and local x-ray and magnetic resonance imaging or CT. Needle biopsies may be appropriate and can often be done in the radiology suite. A venous access port is appropriate only if the diagnosis of a cancer is established.
Textbook: Page 521 ANSWER: B

22. Which bone tumors are radiographic diagnoses and don't require biopsy?

A. Chondrosarcoma.
B. Metastasis.
C. Giant cell tumor.
D. Osteochondroma.

DISCUSSION: Chondrosarcoma needs a biopsy for staging purposes; metastasis should be documented the first time it occurs in bone; and giant cell tumor is typically aggressive and requires biopsy and treatment. Osteochondroma can be monitored clinically and radiographically in most instances, obviating the need for a biopsy.
Textbook: Page 519 ANSWER: D

23. Impending fractures should be treated by:

A. Radiation therapy.
B. Chemotherapy.
C. Internal fixation.
D. Bisphosphonates.

DISCUSSION: The mechanical deficiency in a bone with an impending fracture can only be addressed in a timely fashion by surgically reinforcing the bone. Bisphosphonates may prevent further bone loss, but they don't overcome the existing bone weakness. Chemotherapy and radiation therapy are warranted for long-term local and systemic cancer control, but they don't solve the acute mechanical problem.
Textbook: Page 527 ANSWER: C

24. The effectiveness of preoperative chemotherapy for osteogenic sarcoma is:

A. Needed to perform limb-preserving surgery.
B. Predictive of disease-free survival.
C. Useful to tailor postoperative chemotherapy.
D. Determined by the translocation type causing the tumor.

DISCUSSION: Limb preservation can be done without preoperative chemotherapy. Tailoring of chemotherapy has not been successful, despite its inherent appeal. Ewing's sarcoma, not osteogenic sarcoma, is caused by a translocation.
Textbook: Page 525 ANSWER: B

25. Joint replacement to reconstruct defects after a tumor resection is:

A. As successful as after removal of an arthritic joint.
B. Not possible in children under 10 years of age.
C. Best for benign tumor cases.
D. Able to be combined with allograft bone transplantation.

DISCUSSION: Tumor megaprostheses have high failure rates due to septic and aseptic loosening. Expandable prostheses are available now for young children, but the prosthetic revision rate is high. Benign tumors rarely need to be resected or need a joint replacement—most can be treated by intralesional means.
Textbook: Page 523 ANSWER: D

NOTES

NOTES

CHAPTER 8

HEAD AND NECK

1. The combined effects of smoking and alcohol result in numerous genetic mutations. Which of the following mutations has been most commonly found in genetic analysis of head and neck squamous cell carcinoma of the upper aerodigestive tract?

A. p21.
B. p16.
C. p53.
D. H-*ras*.
E. K-*ras*.

DISCUSSION: Although there are numerous gene mutations, and chromosomal deletions and translocations that occur in squamous cell carcinoma of the head and neck, mutations of the tumor suppressor gene p53 have been reported in 40 to 50% of these mucosally derived tumors. In histologically normal mucosal biopsies adjacent to invasive squamous cell carcinoma of the oral cavity and oropharynx, p53 mutations have been identified. It is hypothesized that mutations in this tumor suppressor gene may be an early event in the carcinogenic cascade.

Textbook: Page 534 ANSWER: C

2. The concept of field cancerization signifies which of the following?

A. The tendency for epithelial neoplasms to spread centrifugally from the initial nidus of neoplasia.
B. The induction of second malignancies in a previously irradiated region.
C. Simultaneous malignancies of the genitourinary system and oral cavity.
D. Multiple genetic and epigenetic events occurring throughout the upper aerodigestive tract following long-term exposure to carcinogens with subsequent development of multiple primary tumors.
E. Tumor microemboli that spread throughout the submucosal lymphatics to produce "drop metastases."

DISCUSSION: In chemical carcinogenesis, multiple genetic events occur in the basal cell layer of the mucosa of the upper aerodigestive tract. The principal carcinogens involved with tumor oogenesis are tobacco smoke and alcohol. Alcohol serves as a promoter to the carcinogenic effects of tobacco. In sites of the upper aerodigestive tract where the basal cell layer of the mucosa comes in contact with these carcinogenic agents, multiple genetic events may occur which, over time, predispose to expression of the malignant phenotype. Throughout the oral cavity, oropharynx, esophagus, and lung, these genetic events may produce the emergence of multiple primary tumors. Among patients with a squamous cell carcinoma of the upper aerodigestive tract, the incidence of a simultaneous second primary tumor is 2 to 3%. Synchronous multiple primary tumors (found within 6 months of the initial diagnosis) may be found in 10% of patients. Metachronous tumors are those that arise more than 6 months after the initial diagnosis of the primary tumor. Following the diagnosis of the index head and neck cancer, the risk for the development of metachronous primary tumors in the upper aerodigestive tract, lung, and esophagus is approximately 10% per year.

Textbook: Page 534 ANSWER: D

3. Elective treatment of cervical lymphatics should be considered when the risk of occult metastatic disease within cervical lymph nodes is:

A. 5%.
B. 10%.
C. 15%.
D. 20%.
E. 50%.

DISCUSSION: It has been recommended that the regional lymphatics should be treated among patients with a squamous carcinoma of the upper aerodigestive tract if the risk for occult disease in regional lymph nodes is 20% or greater. There are few prospective studies that demonstrate a survival advantage for elective treatment of the neck for patients with upper aerodigestive tract squamous carcinoma. Nevertheless, it has been well documented that for oral tongue cancer the risk of occult metastasis in T1 and T2 primary tumors is 20 to 25%. Studies have demonstrated that elective treatment of the cervical lymphatics by selective neck dissection may provide a survival advantage by clearance of occult metastatic nodal disease as opposed to a watch-and-wait approach.

Textbook: Page 536 ANSWER: D

4. Referred pain to the ear is frequently seen with carcinomas arising from the:

A. Lower gum.
B. Maxillary sinus.

C. Nasopharynx.
D. Base of the tongue.
E. Cervical esophagus.

DISCUSSION: Tumors arising in the base of the tongue frequently produce few symptoms. This is a so-called silent area of the upper aerodigestive tract. Frequently patients present initially with referred pain to the ear. In an individual with otalgia and a history of smoking and alcohol use, the physician should always consider the presence of a primary tumor in the base of the tongue or pharynx when the ear examination is normal.

Textbook: Page 539 ANSWER: D

NOTES

NOTES

CHAPTER 9

BREAST

1. A 56-year-old woman with Stage I infiltrating ductal carcinoma of the right breast desires immediate breast reconstruction without the use of implants. She wears a 46D cup bra with Grade II ptosis. She smokes one pack of cigarettes a day and is approximately 25 pounds overweight. Which of the following flaps is the most appropriate for immediate breast reconstruction?

A. Latissimus dorsi myocutaneous flap.
B. Single pedicle transverse rectus abdominis myocutaneous (TRAM) flap.
C. Free TRAM flap.
D. Tissue expander and permanent implant.

DISCUSSION: A large-volume reconstruction, both in terms of skin envelope and subcutaneous fill, is needed, precluding use of the smaller skin envelope of the expander or latissimus dorsi. The smoking history is a relative contraindication to a pedicle TRAM flap.

Textbook: Page 597 ANSWER: C

2. A pedicle transverse rectus abdominis myocutaneous (TRAM) flap cannot be used for breast reconstruction in the patient who has had which of the following abdominal procedures?

A. Appendectomy.
B. Laparoscopic cholecystectomy.
C. C-section transverse incision.
D. Abdominoplasty.

DISCUSSION: Abdominoplasty lifts the overlying skin and severs the blood supply from the underlying rectus abdominis muscles. None of the other incisions listed cut across the muscle pedicle.

Textbook: Page 597 ANSWER: D

3. A 49-year-old woman with a T4 breast carcinoma adherent to the chest wall is advised to undergo a radical mastectomy followed by a course of radiation therapy. Which of the possible types of breast reconstruction is contraindicated?

A. Latissimus dorsi musculocutaneous flap, without implant.
B. Single pedicle transverse rectus abdominis myocutaneous (TRAM) flap.
C. Free TRAM flap.
D. Placement of a tissue expander, followed by placement of a permanent implant.

DISCUSSION: Although capsular contracture may occur around an implant, radiation treatment causes fibrosis which makes tissue expansion almost impossible. Moreover, the resulting ischemia results in a significantly higher rate of expander exposure and extrusion. The autogenous flaps listed may become fibrotic and even involute to an extent. However, they are considered safer alternatives to tissue expansion.

Textbook: Page 595 ANSWER: D

4. A 48-year-old woman who is an avid golfer and swimmer is diagnosed with a Stage I breast carcinoma. Which of the following options is most likely to have an impact on her lifestyle by limiting function?

A. Pedicle transverse rectus abdominis myocutaneous (TRAM) flap.
B. Tissue expansion followed by permanent implant.
C. Latissimus dorsi musculocutaneous flap, with implant.
D. Inferior gluteus maximus free flap.

DISCUSSION: The latissimus dorsi muscle assists in elevation of the arm. Consequently, it is an important muscle for back swing in golf or in tennis. This patient's active lifestyle would be significantly impinged by the loss of one of these muscles. The other methods of reconstruction would not significantly impair her daily activity or her avocations.

Textbook: Page 596 ANSWER: C

5. Immmediate breast reconstruction (performed at the same time as the mastectomy):

A. Obscures detection of local recurrence.
B. Is more costly.
C. Yields poorer quality results.
D. Has fewer complications.
E. Causes a slower return to work.

DISCUSSION: Immediate breast reconstruction is performed immediately following the ablative mastectomy at the same operative setting. Studies have shown that reconstruction does not obscure the detection of local recurrence. The complication rate is greater than for mastectomy alone, but less than for separate-setting (delayed) mastectomy and reconstruction. The same is true for the cost and the duration of postoperative disability.

Textbook: Page 599 ANSWER: D

6. After intraductal papilloma, unilateral bloody nipple discharge from one duct orifice is most commonly caused by which of the following pathologic conditions?

A. Paget's disease of the nipple.
B. Intraductal carcinoma.
C. Inflammatory carcinoma.
D. Subareolar mastitis.

DISCUSSION: Nipple discharge is surgically significant when it is grossly bloody and when it appears at a single duct orifice on one nipple. Bloody discharge is usually due to a benign intraductal papilloma; however, intraductal carcinoma in the large ducts under the nipple can be the cause of bloody discharge, and pathologically the lesion is frequently a large papillary tumor that has become malignant. Paget's disease of the nipple is also due to intraductal carcinoma arising in subareolar ducts, but it rarely is associated with nipple discharge. Subareolar mastitis may produce nipple discharge, but it is purulent and not bloody. Inflammatory carcinoma is not associated with nipple discharge.

Textbook: Page 559 ANSWER: B

7. Which of the following conditions is associated with increased risk of breast cancer?

A. Fibrocystic mastopathy.
B. Severe hyperplasia.
C. Atypical hyperplasia.
D. Papillomatosis.

DISCUSSION: Fibrocystic mastopathy, or fibrocystic disease, was once thought to increase the risk of breast cancer; however, later studies of the pathologic findings in fibrocystic complex found an increased cancer risk only for patients whose biopsies showed atypical hyperplasia. "Severe hyperplasia" is a pathologic term that refers to the amount of hyperplasia and is frequently seen in the biopsy specimens of young women; it is a misleading term and is not associated with a disease risk. Papillomatosis is also part of the fibrocystic complex and is a frequent finding in benign breast biopsies; it does not confer an increased risk of cancer.

Textbook: Page 561 ANSWER: C

8. Which of the following breast lesions are noninvasive malignancies?

A. Intraductal carcinoma of the comedo type.
B. Tubular carcinoma and mucinous carcinoma.
C. Infiltrating ductal carcinoma and lobular carcinoma.
D. Medullary carcinoma, including atypical medullary lesions.

DISCUSSION: Tubular, mucinous, and medullary carcinomas are histologic variants of infiltrating ductal cancer and are all invasive malignancies. Infiltrating lobular cancer is a particular histologic variant of invasive breast cancer characterized by permeation of the stroma with small cells that resemble those found in the breast lobule or acinus. Intraductal carcinoma refers to a malignancy of ductal origin that remains enclosed within duct structures. This noninvasive proliferation can undergo central necrosis, which frequently calcifies to form the microcalcifications seen on mammography. The central necrosis within enlarged and back-to-back ductal structures resembles comedoes and gives rise to the term "comedo-carcinoma," now reserved for this histologic variety of intraductal carcinoma.

Textbook: Page 570 ANSWER: A

9. Which of the following are the most important and clinically useful risk factors for breast cancer?

A. Fibrocystic disease, age, and gender.
B. Cysts, family history in immediate relatives, and gender.
C. Age, gender, and family history in immediate relatives.
D. Obesity, nulliparity, and alcohol use.

DISCUSSION: The most important risk factors for breast cancer are the patient's age, gender, and a family history of breast cancer in immediate relatives (sisters, mother, daughter). The age-adjusted incidence of breast cancer increases with age. Breast cancer does occur in males, but the disease is far more common in women. Family history is important when breast cancer occurs within the immediate family; history of breast cancer in more distant relatives (grandmothers, cousins, aunts) is less important. In addition, age factors into the risk associated with family history. An affected young primary relative is far more significant as a risk factor than an older relative with breast cancer. The other important risk factor not listed here is a history of breast cancer, either within the conserved ipsilateral breast or in the contralateral breast. Again, age plays an important modifying role; as the age at which breast cancer was first diagnosed increases, the risk of a subsequent second cancer decreases. Although patients with fibrocystic disease are at increased risk for breast cancer, risk concentrates in those patients with fibrocystic disease who show atypical epithelial hyperplasia within breast ducts. Obesity, nulliparity, and alcohol all appear to increase risk slightly and are important to the epidemiologic study of breast cancer; however, the effect of these factors is not sufficient to warrant their consideration in common clinical practice.

Textbook: Page 561 ANSWER: C

10. Which of the following pathologic findings is the strongest contraindication to breast preservation (lumpectomy with breast radiation) as primary treatment for a newly diagnosed breast cancer?

A. Grade 3, poorly differentiated, infiltrating ductal carcinoma.
B. Extensive intraductal cancer around the invasive lesion.
C. Tumor size greater than 3 cm.
D. Positive surgical margin for invasive cancer.

DISCUSSION: The only firm contraindication to wide excision and radiation (breast preservation, lumpectomy) as the primary surgical treatment for a newly discovered breast cancer is the inability to achieve an uninvolved surgical margin after excision of the tumor. A positive surgical margin requires, at least, reoperation with an attempt at re-excision of the cancer. If the margin of removal is positive after attempts at re-excision, this is a strong reason to recommend mastectomy in preference to breast conservation. Tumor size is a relative contraindication when the cancer is so large in relation to the breast that excision to a clean surgical margin seems unreasonable. Other histologic findings, such as tumor grade or vascular invasion, are not strong reasons to recommend mastectomy if the patient would prefer breast conservation.

Textbook: Page 577 ANSWER: D

11. The proper treatment for lobular carcinoma in situ (LCIS) includes which of the following components?

A. Close follow-up.
B. Radiation after excision.
C. Mirror-image biopsy of the opposite breast.
D. Mastectomy and regional node dissection.

DISCUSSION: LCIS is best thought of as a precursor lesion that confers increased risk for eventual cancer. The magnitude of this risk appears to be in the range of seven- to ninefold over baseline risk. The chance of breast cancer is equal in both breasts, not just in the biopsied breast, and the type of cancer is not confined to a lobular histology. After a diagnosis of LCIS, patients are at increased risk for invasive and noninvasive ductal carcinoma in both breasts. Therefore, mirror-image biopsy as practiced in the past has little to offer. Since LCIS is purely noninvasive, nodal dissection is not required if mastectomy is chosen. There are no data on the use of breast radiation therapy for LCIS. Most surgical oncologists recommend close follow-up for patients who have LCIS only; the alternative surgical treatment that makes most sense is bilateral simple mastectomies, with or without reconstruction.

Textbook: Page 581 ANSWER: A

12. Which of the following statements most accurately reflects the findings of large overview analyses of clinical trials in which adjuvant chemotherapy for early-stage breast cancer was compared to a control group treated only with surgery?

A. The benefit of adjuvant therapy is confined to young patients.
B. Adjuvant therapy benefits all patients and is independent of age or node status.
C. Adjuvant therapy does not work in estrogen-positive patients.
D. The magnitude of benefit is very large.

DISCUSSION: An overview analysis (meta-analysis) examined nearly all randomized clinical trials in which chemotherapy after surgery was compared to surgery alone for treatment of early-stage breast cancer. This examination of the world's published literature revealed that the magnitude of benefit (the reduction in the odds of recurrence) from chemotherapy was relatively small and in the range of a 20% reduction in the chance of recurrence or death; however, this benefit extended to patients of all ages (young and older) and to both node-positive and node-negative patients. The value of adjuvant chemotherapy does not depend on the hormone receptor content of the cancer. It is useful to remember that a constant reduction in the odds of recurrence results in a higher absolute benefit as the prognosis worsens. If the chance of recurrence is 50% (for node-positive groups) the absolute reduction will be in the range of 10% or 15%. In contrast, if the recurrence rate is 10%, the absolute difference between treated and control groups will be less than 5%. This means that many patients need to be exposed to the risks and side effects of chemotherapy to benefit a very small number. This kind of thinking is currently used to decide who should receive adjuvant chemotherapy after primary treatment (mastectomy or lumpectomy).

Textbook: Page 588 ANSWER: B

NOTES

NOTES

NOTES

CHAPTER 10

ENDOCRINE

1. Surgery of a chronically inflamed thyroglossal duct cyst requires:

A. Chronic antibiotic therapy prior to surgical removal.
B. Removal of the central portion of the hyoid bone.
C. Division of the sternothyroid muscle.
D. Adequate drainage.
E. Identification of the recurrent laryngeal nerve.

DISCUSSION: The chronically inflamed thyroglossal duct cyst requires complete removal for cure. Because of the embryologic derivation of this midline deformity, the entire track up to and including the central portion of the hyoid bone needs to be removed. The track then proceeds superiorly to the base of the tongue. If this entire track (including the central portion of the hyoid bone) is not removed, then recurrence and recurrent infection can occur. The recurrent laryngeal nerve need not be identified, as the surgery is entirely midline. Likewise, strap muscles do not need to be divided. Adequate drainage and chronic antibiotic therapy prior to surgical removal, although good principles for local control of an infectious process, are not the main principles of surgical excision.

Textbook: Page 604 ANSWER: B

2. Which of the following is the most reasonable biochemical marker to follow after total thyroidectomy for papillary carcinoma?

A. Calcitonin.
B. Ionized calcium.
C. Serum thyroid-stimulating hormone.
D. Carcinoembryonic antigen.
E. Thyroglobulin.

DISCUSSION: Thyroglobulin is the most reasonable marker to follow after total thyroidectomy. Thyroglobulin is a glycoprotein that is produced only by normal or neoplastic thyroid follicular cells. Thyroglobulin levels should fall to zero after total thyroidectomy, and any detectable levels after thyroidectomy should be due to neoplastic tissues, thereby predicting recurrence. The other markers are not associated with predictable evidence of recurrence for papillary carcinoma.

Textbook: Page 607 ANSWER: E

3. The action of steroid in hyperthyroid patients is to:

A. Block peripheral conversion of thyroxin (T_4) to triiodothyronine (T_3).
B. Inhibit uptake of inorganiciodide by thyroid.
C. Enhance metabolism of peripheral T_4.
D. Block thyrotropin-releasing hormone (TRH) release.
E. Inhibit uptake of inorganic iodide by the gastrointestinal tract.

DISCUSSION: Steroid therapy for the hyperthyroid patient is an important modality through which to gain control of the clinical state of hyperthyroidism. Glucocorticoids can swiftly and rapidly block the peripheral conversion of T_4 to T_3. In addition, steroids may have an effect by blocking the TRH release (however, they do not have an effect on TRH release). The other choices are not affected by steroid administration.

Textbook: Page 608 ANSWER: A

4. The 14-year-old daughter of a known multiple endocrine neoplasia Type 2 (MEN 2) woman presents with a thyroid mass. Of the following tests, which is the most important in terms of future surgical management?

A. Ultrasound-guided fine-needle aspiration (FNA).
B. Twenty-four-hour urinary catecholamine determination.
C. Liver function tests.
D. Chest x-ray.
E. Indirect laryngoscopy.

DISCUSSION: It is very important to measure 24-hour urinary catecholamines in a MEN 2 family because of the incidence of pheochromocytoma. General anesthesia in an undiagnosed pheochromocytoma could result in a devastating clinical situation. The other choices in this question are not completely necessary. Ultrasound-guided FNA might be reasonable for a thyroid mass; however, it does not have a 100% accuracy in diagnosing medullary thyroid cancer.

Textbook: Page 703 ANSWER: B

5. The preferred treatment for a 2.5-cm papillary carcinoma in the right lobe of a 25-year-old woman is:

A. Enucleation.
B. Lobectomy and left lymph node dissection.

C. Total thyroidectomy and right lymph node dissection.
D. Total thyroidectomy and central lymph node dissection.
E. Total thyroidectomy.

DISCUSSION: In this situation total thyroidectomy is the best choice. There is literature suggesting that right thyroid lobectomy and isthmectomy might be a reasonable alternative; however, this is not given as one of the other choices. Enucleation is inadequate, and the rate of recurrence would be high. There is no need for a lymph node dissection in this situation. Any lesion over 1 or 1.5 cm, even in a young woman with a predictably good prognosis, should be treated with total thyroidectomy.

Textbook: Page 618 ANSWER: E

6. Which of the following conditions can be diagnosed with 100% sensitivity and specificity using fine-needle aspiration (FNA)?

A. Medullary cancer.
B. Colloid nodule.
C. Follicular cancer.
D. Anaplastic cancer.
E. Papillary cancer.

DISCUSSION: Fine-needle aspiration is an excellent diagnostic tool particularly for patients with papillary carcinoma. The diagnosis of papillary carcinoma of the thyroid can be made by evaluation of individual cellular pathology. Medullary carcinoma and anaplastic carcinoma are very hard to diagnose with FNA, and the sensitivity, in most large series, is nowhere near 100%. Follicular carcinoma cannot be diagnosed using FNA because documentation of vascular invasion is necessary to make the diagnosis. A colloid nodule can be diagnosed with FNA by demonstrating colloid and macrophage deposition; however, the sensitivity of this diagnosis is not 100%. Therefore, papillary carcinoma is the best answer.

Textbook: Page 615 ANSWER: E

7. Which of the following statements regarding the differential diagnosis of hypercalcemia is correct?

A. Malignant tumors typically cause hypercalcemia by the ectopic production of parathyroid hormone (PTH).
B. The diagnosis of primary hyperparathyroidism is supported by serum levels of calcium of 10.8 mg/dl; chloride, 104 mmol/L; bicarbonate, 21 mmol/L; phosphorus, 2.4 mg/dl and by an elevated PTH level.
C. Familial hypocalciuric hypercalcemia is distinguished from primary hyperparathyroidism based on parathyroid imaging.
D. Although serum albumin binds calcium, the measured total calcium is usually unaffected in patients with severe hypoproteinemia.
E. Thiazide diuretics are a good treatment for hypercalcemia and can be continued in the patient with apparent hypercalcemia of malignancy.

DISCUSSION: Malignant tumors rarely secrete PTH itself; they can secrete parathyroid hormone–related peptide or cytokine activators of osteoclast activity. The diagnosis of primary hyperparathyroidism is supported by hypercalcemia with a mild hyperchloremic metabolic acidosis and a chloride-phosphate ratio greater than 33 or a modified chloride (mmol/L/mg/dl)-phosphate ratio greater than 500. Familial hypercalciuric hypercalcemia is distinguished from primary hyperparathyroidism by a low urine calcium. Serum calcium changes approximately 0.8 mg/dl for every 1 g/dl similar change in serum albumin. Thiazide diuretics can cause hypercalcemia and should not be used in patients who are hypercalcemic.

Textbook: Page 635 ANSWER: B

8. All of the following are indications for operation in a patient with previously asymptomatic hyperparathyroidism, except:

A. Age greater than 60.
B. Nephrolithiasis.
C. A substantial decline in renal function.
D. A substantial decline in bone mass.
E. Depression and fatigue.

DISCUSSION: Age less than 50 is considered an indication for operation. All of the other answers are indications for operation.

Textbook: Page 639 ANSWER: A

9. The parathyroid glands:

A. Develop from the second and third pharyngeal pouches, along with the palatine tonsil and the thymus.
B. Migrate caudally in the neck in normal development, but can be found anywhere from the pharyngeal mucosa to the deep mediastinum.
C. Secrete parathyroid hormone and calcitonin to manage calcium homeostasis.
D. Usually are four in number, but frequently number only two or three.
E. Contain enzymes that catalyze the conversion of 25(OH) vitamin D_3 to $1,25(OH)_2$ vitamin D_3.

DISCUSSION: The parathyroid glands develop from the third and fourth pharyngeal pouches, along with the thymus and the thyroid ultimobronchial body; there are four glands in the vast majority of cases. Calcitonin is secreted by the C cells of the thyroid. Vitamin D_3 hydroxylation occurs in the kidney.

Textbook: Page 629 ANSWER: B

10. Primary hyperparathyroidism can contribute to all of the following health problems, except:

A. Peptic ulcer disease.
B. Acute pancreatitis.
C. Calciphylaxis.
D. Psychosis.
E. Hypertension.

DISCUSSION: Primary hyperparathyroidism can cause a variety of systemic complaints. Gastrointestinal involvement includes pancreatitis and peptic ulcer disease. The kidneys can be affected by nephrocalcinosis or nephrolithiasis. The bones can be severely affected by bone resorption. Neuromuscular complaints can include weakness and fatigue, as well as psychosis. Hypertension is present in as many as 70% of individuals with hyperparathyroidism, and may be related to the renal disease. Calciphylaxis (soft tissue necrosis with calcium deposits) is a feature of renal osteodystrophy rather than primary hyperparathyroidism.

Textbook: Page 538 ANSWER: C

11. Secondary hyperparathyroidism:

A. Is a metabolic disease in which the primary abnormality is an independent overproduction of parathyroid hormone by one or more parathyroid glands.
B. Is best treated initially by subtotal parathyroidectomy.
C. Is caused by increased production of 1,25$(OH)_2$ vitamin D_3, causing increasing intestinal calcium absorption and hypercalcemia.
D. Can have severe effects on bones exacerbated by aluminum contained in phosphate binders and dialysate water.
E. Is best treated initially by total parathyroidectomy with autotransplantation.

DISCUSSION: Secondary hyperparathyroidism is caused by renal disease, including decreased glomerular filtration rate and decreased 1,25$(OH)_2$ vitamin D_3 production. It is best treated by medical management restricting dietary phosphate, administering vitamin D and calcium with phosphate binding gels, and limiting aluminum exposure, which can exacerbate bone disease.

Textbook: Page 638 ANSWER: D

12. All of the following are true of hypoparathyroidism, except:

A. It is most commonly encountered as a post-viral syndrome.
B. It can be associated with marked hypocalcemia after parathyroidectomy in patients with bone disease.
C. It can cause anxiety, depression, or confusion.
D. It can cause physical signs such as Chvostek's and Trousseau's signs.
E. It is treatable acutely with intravenous calcium salts, and chronically with oral calcium and vitamin D.

DISCUSSION: Hypoparathyroidism is most commonly encountered after thyroid surgery. It can temporarily be severe after parathroidectomy in patients with bone disease ("postoperative bone hunger"). The signs and symptoms can include anxiety, depression, confusion, Chvostek's sign and Trousseau's sign, as well as circumoral or extremity tingling, and tetany with carpopedal spasms or seizures. Treatment is as noted.

Textbook: Page 644 ANSWER: A

13. Sestamibi scan for the localization of abnormal parathyroid tissue:

A. Is useful to confirm the diagnosis of hyperparathyroidism in the equivocal situation.
B. Is mandatory before initial neck exploration for primary hyperparathyroidism.
C. Can localize ectopic abnormal parathyroid tissue in patients with persistent hyperparathyroidism.
D. Can be used to select patients who might benefit from parathyroidectomy.
E. Images the abnormal parathyroid glands in greater than 95% of patients with hyperparathyroidism.

DISCUSSION: Hyperparathyroidism is a biochemical diagnosis that should be clear-cut before any imaging tests are considered. The standard approach to neck exploration for hyperparathyroidism does not require preoperative imaging. The indications for operation in a patient with hyperparathyroidism should not be based on the presence of imageable parathyroid tissue. Sestamibi scanning demonstrates abnormal parathyroid glands in 70 to 85% of patients, depending on the selected population.

Textbook: Page 639 ANSWER: C

14. The endocrine tumor of the pancreas with the lowest rate of malignancy is:

A. Glucagonoma.
B. Somatostatinoma.
C. Gastrinoma.
D. Insulinoma.
E. VIPoma.

DISCUSSION: The endocrine tumor of the pancreas with the lowest rate of malignancy is insulinoma, which is usually given as 10%, although even that seems high. The hyperinsulinism of metastatic insulinomas can usually be treated medically by octreotide or diazoxide.

Textbook: Page 647 ANSWER: D

15. Which of the following actions is not performed by insulin?

A. Decreasing blood sugar.
B. Decreasing protein synthesis.
C. Decreasing glycogenolysis.
D. Decreasing lipolysis.
E. Increasing glucose transport.

DISCUSSION: Insulin stores energy by decreasing blood sugar, *increasing* protein synthesis, decreasing glycogenolysis, decreasing lipolysis, and increasing glucose transport into cells, fulfilling its role as the hormone of energy storage.

Textbook: Page 649 ANSWER: B

16. The best means to localize a gastrinoma preoperatively is:

A. Enhanced magnetic resonance imaging.
B. Selective portal venous sampling.
C. Calcium angiography.
D. Somatostatin receptor scintigraphy.
E. Endoscopic ultrasound.

DISCUSSION: The best means to localize a gastrinoma preoperatively is by somatostatin receptor scintigraphy. Selective portal venous sampling is not as helpful in gastrinomas as it is in insulinomas, and calcium angiography is one of the methods of choice for localizing an insulinoma but is not as helpful with gastrin-producing tumors. The high degree of sensitivity of somatostatin receptor scintigraphy renders it the test of choice.

Textbook: Page 655 ANSWER: D

17. Of the following, the best preoperative method for localization of insulinoma is:

A. Somatostatin receptor scintigraphy.
B. Enhanced magnetic resonance imaging.
C. Spiral computed tomography.
D. Selective portal venous sampling.
E. Secretin arteriography.

DISCUSSION: The technique of selective arterial injection of calcium (calcium angiography) holds promise, but at present the best results are gathered by inserting a catheter transhepatically into the portal vein and then into the splenic vein, withdrawing and taking serial samples, noting the position of the sample obtained.

Textbook: Page 651 ANSWER: D

18. Of endocrine tumors of the pancreas, the best prognosis for cure is in:

A. Insulinoma.
B. Somatostatinoma.
C. VIPoma.
D. Glucagonoma.
E. Gastrinoma.

DISCUSSION: Insulinoma has a 10% risk of mortality, and the incidence of metastases in all the other endocrine tumors mentioned is at least 50%.

Textbook: Page 653 ANSWER: A

19. The most effective intraoperative technique for localizing a pancreatic gastrinoma involves palpation plus:

A. Intraoperative endoscopy with transillumination.
B. Selective venous sampling.
C. Intra-arterial injection of vital-blue dye.
D. Intraoperative ultrasonography.
E. Caudal pancreatectomy.

DISCUSSION: In experienced hands, intraoperative ultrasonography has proved highly effective.

Textbook: Page 656 ANSWER: D

20. Hormones released by the posterior pituitary, or neurohypophysis, include:

A. Prolactin.
B. Thyroid-stimulating hormone.
C. Cortisol.
D. Oxytocin.
E. Luteinizing hormone.

DISCUSSION: The posterior pituitary, or neurohypophysis, includes the posterior lobe, the pituitary stalk, and the median eminence of the pituitary. Antidiuretic hormone and oxytocin are synthesized in the hypothalamus and transported through axons to the posterior pituitary, where the active hormones are released into the circulation. Prolactin, thyroid-stimulating hormone, and luteinizing hormone are made by cells of the anterior pituitary. Cortisol is made by and secreted by the adrenal cortex.

Textbook: Page 663 ANSWER: D

21. Which of the following hormones is not made by cells of the anterior pituitary?

A. Prolactin.
B. Follicle-stimulating hormone.
C. Antidiuretic hormone (ADH).
D. Adrenocorticotropic hormone.
E. Growth hormone.

DISCUSSION: ADH and oxytocin are made by the hypothalamus and transported down axons to the posterior pituitary, where they are released into the circulation. Prolactin, follicle-stimulating hormone, adrenocorticotropic hormone, growth hormone, luteinizing hormone, prolactin, and thyroid-stimulating hormone are released by the anterior pituitary.

Textbook: Page 665 ANSWER: C

22. The following statements about antidiuretic hormone (ADH) are true except:

A. ADH is a nine-amino-acid peptide hormone derived from the same ancestral hormone as vasopressin.
B. ADH is secreted in response to a rise in plasma osmolality less than 285 mOsm.
C. ADH secretion is inhibited by alcohol, lithium, and phenytoin.
D. ADH is secreted in conjunction with angiotensin II.
E. ADH stimulates sodium and chloride reabsorption by cells of the ascending loop of Henle.

DISCUSSION: All of the above statements are correct except for statement D. ADH is secreted from the posterior pituitary in conjunction with neurophysin II.

Textbook: Page 665 ANSWER: D

23. Diabetes insipidus is caused by deficiency of:

A. Antidiuretic hormone (ADH).
B. Renin.
C. Angiotensin II.

D. Insulin.
E. Oxytocin.

DISCUSSION: Diabetes insipidus is characterized by prolonged polyuria and polydipsia, and is confirmed by a combination of high plasma osmolality (>285 mOsm) and low urine osmolality (<285 mOsm). It is caused by a deficiency of ADH.

Textbook: Page 665 ANSWER: A

24. The following statements regarding prolactinomas are true except:

A. Prolactinomas are the most common functional pituitary tumors.
B. Prolactinomas occur in up to 40% of patients with multiple endocrine neoplasia Type 1 syndrome.
C. Prolactin hypersecretion may cause hypogonadism, galactorrhea, and amenorrhea.
D. Prolactinomas should be treated by transsphenoidal resection.
E. Bromocriptine is the preferred treatment for prolactinomas.

DISCUSSION: Although surgery was previously routinely recommended for treatment of prolactinomas, bromocriptine is now the preferred treatment for patients with prolactin-secreting micro- and macroadenomas, and for patients with large, invasive prolactinomas. Because bromocriptine treatment is lifelong and expensive, some patients opt for surgical resection by the transsphenoidal approach.

Textbook: Page 668 ANSWER: D

25. Diagnostic work-up of the patient with suspected acromegaly should include all of the following except:

A. High-resolution magnetic resonance imaging of the pituitary with gadolinium enhancement.
B. Measurement of serum insulin-like growth factor-1 (IGF-1) concentration.
C. Testing for glucose suppression of growth hormone (GH) release.
D. Measurement of serum calcium.
E. Measurement of plasma calcitonin level.

DISCUSSION: Measurement of random GH levels is extremely variable and is not helpful in the diagnosis of GH excess. Measurement of serum IGF-1 is a useful screening test, and demonstration of elevated GH levels following administration of glucose is confirmatory. Because GH-producing adenomas may occur in multiple endocrine neoplasia Type 1, calcium levels should be measured. Calcitonin is secreted by medullary thyroid carcinomas, which are a feature of multiple endocrine neoplasia Type 2 (MEN 2). Pituitary tumors are not a feature of MEN 2.

Textbook: Page 669 ANSWER: E

26. Effective treatments for growth hormone–producing pituitary adenomas include all of the following except:

A. Transfrontal resection.
B. Transsphenoidal resection.
C. Octreotide.
D. Bromocriptine.
E. External-beam radiation therapy.

DISCUSSION: Transsphenoidal resection is the treatment of choice for growth hormone–producing pituitary microadenomas and macroadenomas. For larger tumors that have transgressed the diaphragma sella into the subarachnoid space, transfrontal resection may be necessary. External-beam radiation therapy is given for residual tumors in cases of incomplete resection, and may be used as primary therapy in some patients at high surgical risk. Panhypopituitarism occurs in 50% of patients following pituitary irradiation. Octreotide may shrink larger tumors when given preoperatively, and may be effective in patients with residual disease after incomplete resection. Bromocriptine is effective treatment for prolactinomas.

Textbook: Page 670 ANSWER: D

27. Extra-adrenal pheochromocytomas predominantly secrete:

A. Epinephine.
B. Norepinephrine.
C. Dopamine.
D. Vanillylmandelic acid.
E. Metanephrine.

DISCUSSION: In adrenal chromaffin tissue, the enzyme phenylethanolamine-*N*-methyl transferase (PMNT) converts norepinephrine to epinephrine. Extra-adrenal chromaffin tissue lacks this enzyme, and thus secretes predominantly norepinephrine. Epinephrine and norepinephrine are metabolized in the liver and kidney to vanillylmandelic acid, metanephrine, and normetanephrine.

Textbook: Page 685 ANSWER: B

28. Aldosterone is synthesized and secreted in the adrenal by cells of the:

A. Zona reticularis.
B. Zona fasciculata.
C. Zona glomerulosa.
D. Adrenal medulla.

DISCUSSION: The adrenal cortex is composed of three layers: the zona reticularis, the zona fasciculata, and the zona glomerulosa. Glucocorticoids and adrenal androgens are synthesized in the inner zona fasciculata and zona reticularis. Mineralocorticoids (aldosterone) are secreted in the outer zona glomerulosa. The adrenal medulla secretes catecholamines.

Textbook: Page 677 ANSWER: C

29. The combination of masculinization and Cushing's syndrome in a woman is highly suggestive of:

A. Adrenocorticotropic hormone (ACTH)–producing pituitary adenoma.
B. Congenital adrenal hyperplasia.

C. Ectopic ACTH syndrome.
D. Adrenocortical carcinoma.
E. Nelson's syndrome.

DISCUSSION: Excess production of adrenal androgens (dehydroepiandrosterone and androstenedione) by an adenoma or adrenocortical carcinoma may produce virilization in females, and is often associated with Cushing's syndrome, due to associated overproduction of glucocorticoids. Ectopic ACTH syndrome and ACTH-producing pituitary adenomas (Cushing's disease) produce Cushing's syndrome, and do not generally cause virilization. Congenital adrenal hyperplasia is caused by inherited defects in one or more of the enzymes necessary for cortisol biosynthesis, and results in cortisol deficiency. Nelson's syndrome is the development of an ACTH-producing pituitary tumor following bilateral adrenalectomy for Cushing's disease.

Textbook: Page 682 ANSWER: D

30. The diagnosis of primary hyperaldosteronism includes demonstration of all of the following except:

A. Elevated aldosterone level that fails to suppress with volume depletion.
B. Hypokalemia.
C. Elevated urinary potassium.
D. Suppressed plasma renin activity in the face of volume depletion.
E. Elevated serum cortisol levels.

DISCUSSION: In primary aldosteronism, release of inappropriately high levels of aldosterone results in retention of sodium and excretion of potassium and hydrogen ion by the kidney. This results in hypertension without edema, and hypokalemia. Adrenal imaging studies demonstrate an adenoma in the majority of patients. Cortisol levels are generally normal in these patients.

Textbook: Page 678 ANSWER: E

31. Clinical signs and symptoms of adrenocortical insufficiency (addisonian crisis) include all of the following except:

A. Hypotension.
B. Fever.
C. Abdominal pain.
D. Nausea and vomiting.
E. Hypertension.

DISCUSSION: Fever is present in approximately 70% of patients with adrenocortical insufficiency, and is the most commonly noted clinical sign of this disorder. Nausea and vomiting are also very common. Hyponatremia, lethargy, abdominal pain, and hypotension occur in slightly less than half of these patients. Hypertension is not a characteristic finding.

Textbook: Page 683 ANSWER: E

32. Extra-adrenal chromaffin tissue may be found in all of the following areas except:

A. Urinary bladder.
B. Organ of Zuckerkandl.
C. Cervical sympathetic chain.
D. Enteric plexus.
E. Posterior mediastinum.

DISCUSSION: Extra-adrenal chromaffin tissue may exist anywhere along the path of neural crest cell migration. This includes the cervical and mediastinal sympathetic ganglia, and anywhere near the heart, aorta, or urinary bladder. This tissue is not found in the enteric plexus.

Textbook: Page 687 ANSWER: D

33. Pheochromocytomas occur in each of the following inherited syndromes except:

A. Multiple endocrine neoplasia Type 2A (MEN 2A).
B. Multiple endocrine neoplasia Type 1 (MEN 1).
C. Von Hippel–Lindau syndrome.
D. Neurofibromatosis Type 1.
E. Multiple endocrine neoplasia Type 2B (MEN 2B).

DISCUSSION: MEN 2A is characterized by the predisposition to development of medullary thyroid carcinoma (MTC), hyperparathyroidism, and pheochromocytomas. In MEN 2B, patients develop MTC and pheochromocytomas, but not hyperparathyroidism. MEN 2B patients also have a characteristic body habitus, megacolon, and mucosal ganglioneuromas. In von Hippel–Lindau disease, patients develop retinal hemangioblastomas; cysts of the kidney, liver, and pancreas; renal carcinoma; and pheochromocytomas. Neurofibromatosis Type 1 is characterized by multiple neurofibromas, café-au-lait spots, and occasionally pheochromocytomas. MEN 1 is characterized by hyperparathyroidism, pancreatic endocrine tumors, and pituitary adenomas. MEN 1 patients may develop adrenocortical adenomas, but not pheochromocytomas.

Textbook: Page 685 ANSWER: B

34. Initial work-up of a patient with an adrenal incidentaloma (adrenal mass discovered incidentally during imaging studies done for another reason) should include all the following except:

A. Serum potassium measurement.
B. Evaluation for hypercortisolism.
C. Twenty-four-hour urine for catecholamines.
D. Needle biopsy.
E. Measurement of blood pressure.

DISCUSSION: Adrenal incidentalomas are found in 3 to 9% of abdominal computed tomography and magnetic resonance imaging scans done for other reasons. Work-up should be aimed at determining if the lesion is functional or if it is malignant. Most incidentalomas are benign, nonfunctional adenomas that may be safely observed. The most common *functional* adrenal tumors are pheochromocytomas, and aldosterone- and cortisol-producing adenomas. All patients with an adrenal incidentaloma should undergo measurement of serum potassium and blood pressure (to screen for aldosteronism), evaluation for hypercortisolism (24-hour urine cortisol measurement or overnight dexamethasone suppression test), and 24-hour urine measurement of catecholamines and metabolites (to screen for pheochromocytoma). Biopsy should *never* be done unless a 24-hour urine measurement for catecholamines has ruled out the presence of a pheochromocytoma, as deaths have been reported from this intervention. Biopsy should be done only in patients with a suspected metastatic lesion, in whom treatment would be altered by the knowledge of adrenal metastasis. If the adrenal incidentaloma is suspicious for a primary adrenal malignancy, it should be resected, not biopsied.

Textbook: Page 688 ANSWER: D

35. A familial form of medullary thyroid carcinoma (MTC) should be suspected whenever:

A. The tumor is multifocal.
B. The tumor is bilateral (foci of tumor are present in both thyroid lobes).
C. Pathologic examination of the resected thyroid gland reveals the presence of C cells.
D. All of the above.

DISCUSSION: Sporadic MTC is unilateral in at least 80% of cases. However, in patients with MTC occurring as a component of the multiple endocrine neoplasia Type 2A or Type 2B syndromes, the tumor is virtually always multifocal and bilateral. Typically, in this setting the MTC appears as multiple whitish-tan tumor nodules in the mid and upper thirds of each thyroid lobe. A diffuse premalignant proliferation of the C cells of the thyroid is thought to precede the development of MTC in patients with familial MTC. This proliferation, known as *C-cell hyperplasia* (CCH), consists of parafollicular clusters of increased numbers of C cells. The finding of CCH in areas of the thyroid adjacent to gross foci of MTC is strong evidence for familial MTC.

Textbook: Page 701 ANSWER: D

36. All of the following are components of the multiple endocrine neoplasia Type 2B (MEN 2B) syndrome except:

A. Multiple neuromas on the lips, tongue, and oral mucosa.
B. Hyperparathyroidism.
C. Medullary thyroid carcinoma (MTC).
D. Pheochromocytoma.

DISCUSSION: MTC and pheochromocytoma occur in both MEN 2A and MEN 2B syndromes. Patients with MEN 2A may also develop hyperplasia of the parathyroid glands. Although some investigators have reported equivocal histologic abnormalities in the parathyroid glands of patients with MEN 2B, hyperparathyroidism is not a component of this syndrome. In contrast to patients with MEN 2A, those with MEN 2B have a characteristic phenotype, including a tall, thin "marfanoid" habitus. Patients with MEN 2B also develop multiple neuromas on the lips, tongue, and oral mucosa, creating the appearance of thick lips.

Textbook: Page 702 ANSWER: B

37. Multiple endocrine neoplasia Type 2A (MEN 2A) and MEN 2B syndromes are associated with germline mutations in the:

A. p53 tumor suppressor gene.
B. H-*ras* gene.
C. N-*myc* gene.
D. *RET* proto-oncogene.

DISCUSSION: Germline mutations in the *RET* proto-oncogene, a receptor tyrosine kinase that maps to chromosome 10, are associated with MEN 2A and MEN 2B syndromes. Homozygous loss of the p53 tumor suppressor gene is associated with the Li-Fraumeni syndrome, and mutations of p53 are present in a variety of human neoplasms. Point mutations in the H-*ras* gene are associated with carcinoma of the colon, lung, and pancreas. Amplification of the N-*myc* gene, when present in neuroblastoma, suggests a poorer prognosis.

Textbook: Page 699 ANSWER: D

38. Which of the following is (are) true concerning islet cell neoplasms of the pancreas in patients with multiple endocrine neoplasia Type 1 (MEN 1)?

A. Islet cell neoplasms in patients with MEN 1 are characteristically multicentric.
B. The most common islet cell neoplasm in patients with MEN 1 is gastrinoma.
C. Islet cell neoplasms in patients with MEN 1 may be malignant.
D. All of the above.

DISCUSSION: The pathologic change in the pancreas of patients with MEN 1 is typically multicentric. Diffuse hyperplasia of islet cells and microadenoma formation are often identified in areas of the gland distant from grossly evident tumor. Tumors are commonly multifocal. Islet cell neoplasms of the pancreas occur in 30 to 80% of patients with MEN 1. The most common islet cell neoplasm in these patients is gastrinoma. Gastrinomas associated with MEN 1 probably account for 20 to 50% of all cases of the Zollinger-Ellison syndrome. The second most common islet cell tumor is insulinoma. Other pancreatic islet cell neoplasms, such as glucagonoma, somatostatinoma, or vasoactive intestinal polypeptide neoplasms (VIPoma), are rarely associated with MEN 1. Approximately 10% of insulinomas and approximately 15% or more of gastrinomas in patients with MEN 1 are malignant.

Textbook: Page 698 ANSWER: D

39. The multiple endocrine neoplasia Type 2 MEN 2 syndromes are characterized by medullary thyroid carcinoma as the principal feature. Recent genetic studies have demonstrated that the MEN 2 syndromes are associated with germline mutations in the:

A. H-*ras* gene.
B. p53 tumor suppressor gene.
C. *RET* proto-oncogene.
D. Tumor suppressor gene.

DISCUSSION: The MEN 2 syndromes are a group of genetically related familial cancer syndromes that are associated with germline mutations in the *RET* proto-oncogene. *RET* is not a tumor suppressor gene. Mutations in the *RET* proto-oncogene have been shown to be dominantly transforming, that is, a mutation in one allelic copy (either inherited in one of the MEN 2 syndromes, or somatically acquired in sporadic medullary thyroid carcinoma) is sufficient for cancer development. Mutations in the H-*ras* oncogene occur with high frequency in a variety of human cancers including lung, pancreas, and follicular thyroid cancers, but are not seen with increased frequency in medullary thyroid cancer. The p53 tumor suppressor gene, which encodes p53, is mutated in a wide variety of human cancers. Germline mutations in p53 result in the Li-Fraumeni syndrome.

Textbook: Page 699 ANSWER: C

40. Local or regional recurrence of medullary thyroid carcinoma (MTC) in the neck is best treated by:

A. Surgery.
B. Radiation therapy.
C. Chemotherapy.
D. Hormonal therapy.

DISCUSSION: In several series, surgery to remove recurrent or residual MTC has been reported to result in significant decreases in calcitonin levels in most patients, and has resulted in some cures. Radiation therapy and chemotherapy have not been shown to result in such decreases in calcitonin levels. There are no long-term data on survival rates in patients treated for recurrent or residual disease.

Textbook: Page 705 ANSWER: A

NOTES

NOTES

CHAPTER 11

GASTROINTESTINAL

1. Which of the following statements about esophageal anatomy is correct?

A. The esophagus has a poor blood supply, which is segmental in distribution and accounts for the high incidence of anastomotic leakage.
B. The esophageal serosa consists of a thin layer of fibroareolar tissue.
C. The esophagus has two distinct muscle layers consisting of an outer, longitudinal layer and an inner, circular layer, which are striated in the upper third and smooth in the distal two thirds.
D. Injury to the recurrent laryngeal nerve results in vocal cord dysfunction but does not affect swallowing.
E. The lymphatic drainage of the esophagus is relatively sparse, localized primarily to adjacent paraesophageal lymph nodes.

DISCUSSION: Poor technique, not poor blood supply, explains most esophageal anastomotic leaks. Although the major blood supply of the esophagus comes from four to six segmental aortic esophageal arteries, there are extensive submucosal collaterals from the inferior thyroid, intercostal, bronchial, inferior phrenic, and left gastric arteries. The esophagus lacks serosa and instead is surrounded by mediastinal connective tissue (adventitia). There are two muscle layers in the esophagus, an outer longitudinal and an inner circular one. Both layers of the upper third of the esophagus consist of striated muscle, while in the lower two thirds they are (nonstriated) smooth muscle. The recurrent laryngeal branches of the vagus nerves provide both parasympathetic innervation to the cervical esophagus and innervation to the upper esophageal sphincter (UES). Injury to the recurrent laryngeal nerve therefore results in improved UES function with secondary aspiration on swallowing as well as vocal cord dysfunction and hoarseness. The esophagus has extensive lymphatic drainage, with lymphatic capillaries coursing longitudinally in the esophageal wall and communicating with paraesophageal, paratracheal and subcarinal, other mediastinal, perigastric, and internal jugular lymph nodes. This accounts for the biologically aggressive nature of esophageal carcinoma, which tends to metastasize early in its course.

Textbook: Page 709 ANSWER: C

2. Which of the following statements about achalasia is correct?

A. In most cases in North America the cause is a parasitic infestation by *Trypanosoma cruzi.*
B. Chest pain and reflux are the usual symptoms.
C. Distal-third esophageal adenocarcinomas may occur in as many as 30% of patients within 10 years of diagnosis.
D. Manometry demonstrates failure of lower esophageal sphincter (LES) relaxation on swallowing and absent or weak simultaneous contractions in the esophageal body after swallowing.
E. Endoscopic botulinum toxin injection of the LES, pneumatic dilatation, and esophagomyotomy provide highly effective curative therapy for achalasia.

DISCUSSION: Although in South America achalasia is the result of Chagas' disease caused by parasitic infestation by the leishmanial forms of *T. cruzi,* in Europe and North America the cause of achalasia is unknown. The common presenting symptoms of achalasia are dysphagia, reflux, and weight loss. Chest pain is an infrequent symptom in achalasia and is more characteristic of esophageal spasm. Achalasia is a premalignant esophageal lesion: the retention esophagitis leads to metaplasia and *squamous cell carcinoma,* which occurs after 15 to 25 years in the middle third of the thoracic esophagus in 10% of patients. The classic manometric findings of achalasia are failure of relaxation of the LES on swallowing and absent or weak simultaneous contractions in the esophageal body after swallowing. Achalasia is currently incurable, and, although endoscopic botulinum toxin injection of the LES, balloon dilatation, and esophagomyotomy effectively relieve dysphagia in the majority of patients, all of these treatments are strictly palliative. The motility disturbance persists throughout life.

Textbook: Page 720 ANSWER: D

3. Which of the following statements regarding the pathology of esophageal carcinoma is correct?

A. Worldwide, adenocarcinoma is the most common esophageal malignancy.
B. Squamous cell carcinoma is most common in the distal esophagus, whereas adenocarcinoma predominates in the middle third.
C. Patients with Barrett's metaplasia are 40 times

more likely than the general population to develop adenocarcinoma.

D. Metastases from esophageal carcinoma are characteristically limited to regional mediastinal lymph nodes adjacent to the tumor.
E. Achalasia, radiation esophagitis, caustic esophageal stricture, and Plummer-Vinson syndrome are all premalignant esophageal lesions that predispose to the development of adenocarcinoma.

DISCUSSION: Histologically, 95% of esophageal cancers worldwide are squamous cell carcinomas, but the incidence of adenocarcinoma is increasing dramatically in the United States and Europe. Squamous cell carcinoma predominates in the upper and middle thirds of the esophagus, whereas adenocarcinoma is the most frequent distal esophageal cancer. A columnar-lined lower esophagus (Barrett's metaplasia) is associated with an incidence of adenocarcinoma approximately 40 times greater than that of the general population. Esophageal cancer is a biologically aggressive tumor that characteristically metastasizes widely to regional and distant lymph nodes as well as to liver and lungs. Recognized premalignant esophageal lesions include achalasia, radiation esophagitis, caustic stricture, Plummer-Vinson syndrome, leukoplakia, esophageal diverticula, and Barrett's metaplasia. All are associated with the development of squamous cell carcinoma.

Textbook: Page 732 ANSWER: C

4. Which of the following statements about the surgical treatment of esophageal carcinoma is correct?

A. The finding of severe dysphagia in association with Barrett's mucosa is an indication for an antireflux operation to prevent subsequent development of carcinoma.
B. Long-term survival at all stages is improved by radical en bloc resection of the esophagus with its contained tumor, adjacent mediastinal tissues, and regional lymph nodes.
C. The morbidity and mortality rates for cervical esophagogastric anastomotic leak are substantially less than those associated with intrathoracic esophagogastric anastomotic leak.
D. The leading complications of transthoracic esophagectomy and intrathoracic esophagogastric anastomosis are bleeding and wound infection.
E. Transhiatal esophagectomy without thoracotomy achieves better long-term survival than transthoracic esophagectomy.

DISCUSSION: Severe dysplasia in Barrett's mucosa is indicative of carcinoma in situ and is an indication for *resectional* therapy, not an antireflux operation. In the majority of patients, local tumor invasion or distant metastases preclude cure when esophageal carcinoma is diagnosed, and attempts to improve survival with a more radical local operation performed in the face of systemic disease have been disappointingly futile. A cervical esophagogastric anastomotic leak causes a relatively minor cervical salivary fistula that heals in 7 to 10 days in 95% of patients. In contrast, an intrathoracic esophagogastric anastomotic leak results in mediastinitis, which is fatal in 50%. The leading complications of transthoracic esophagectomy and an intrathoracic esophagogastric anastomosis are respiratory insufficiency (from combined thoracic and abdominal incisions) and anastomotic leak resulting in mediastinitis and sepsis. Both complications are minimized by transhiatal esophagectomy without thoracotomy plus cervical esophagogastric anastomosis. No single operative approach to the treatment of esophageal cancer has proved superior to others in terms of long-term survival. The biologic behavior of the tumor (its stage and aggressiveness) determines survival.

Textbook: Page 744 ANSWER: C

5. The best management for a 48-hour-old distal esophageal perforation is:

A. Antibiotics and drainage.
B. Division of the esophagus and exclusion of the perforation.
C. Primary repair with buttressing.
D. Resection with cervical esophagostomy, gastrostomy, and jejunostomy.
E. T-tube fistula and drainage.

DISCUSSION: When the esophagus is repaired primarily and covered by well-vascularized autologous tissue, the rates of fistula and death are significantly less than those observed for patients who receive simple repair without any protection. Primary repair with buttressing is the first choice for treatment. Resection is reserved for esophageal perforations with extensive damage to the esophageal wall or with advanced mediastinal infection and sepsis. Exclusion of the perforated esophagus and T-tube drainage of a perforation are alternative approaches that cannot be considered for primary treatment. Antibiotics and drainage as the sole treatment is reserved for a very small, selected population of patients with well-contained esophageal perforation.

Textbook: Page 726 ANSWER: C

6. All of the following contribute to the measured lower esophageal sphincter pressure during stationary esophageal manometry except:

A. Circular muscle fibers of the distal esophagus.
B. Crural fibers of the diaphragm.
C. Pressure gradient between the abdomen and thorax.
D. The phrenoesophageal membrane.

DISCUSSION: The phrenoesophageal membrane does not generate pressure at the distal esophagus. An intact membrane maintains an intra-abdominal portion of the esophagus that contributes to increased pressure due to the gradient between the abdomen and the thorax. Tonic contraction of the distal muscle fibers of the esophagus and the variable pressure generated by the diaphragm during respiration help prevent reflux under normal circumstances and are detected by the manometry catheter.

Textbook: Page 758 ANSWER: D

7. The following are diagnostic of gastroesophageal reflux disease except:

A. Distal acid exposure time of 10% (DeMeester composite score of 45) during a 24-hour pH study.
B. Spontaneous reflux during contrast esophagography (upper gastrointestinal tract barium study).
C. Linear inflammatory ulcers in the distal esophagus.
D. Barrett's esophagus.

DISCUSSION: Spontaneous gastroesophageal reflux is a normal occurrence. This finding on a contrast study is not a reliable indicator of gastroesophageal reflux *disease*. Abnormal acid exposure detected on 24-hour pH monitoring is the gold standard for diagnosing gastroesophageal reflux disease (normal acid exposure in the distal esophagus is <4%, DeMeester composite score should be <14.7). Endoscopic evidence of advanced esophageal injury such as ulcers, strictures, and Barrett's esophagus are diagnostic for reflux disease.

Textbook: Pages 757–759 ANSWER: B

8. Which of the following are true regarding the treatment of gastroesophageal reflux disease?

A. H_2-blockers are as effective as proton pump inhibitors at ameliorating symptoms of reflux.
B. Long-term proton pump inhibitor therapy has been shown to cause gastric cancer in humans.
C. Typical symptoms of reflux improve in 90% of patients undergoing a laparoscopic antireflux procedure.
D. Patients who have no symptom relief from proton pump inhibitor therapy are excellent candidates for operative treatment.

DISCUSSION: Proton pump inhibitors are much more effective at decreasing acid output from parietal cells than are the H_2-blockers. Although proton pump inhibitors are known to induce hyperplastic gastric polyps in some patients, they do not appear to increase the incidence of gastric cancer. Patients who have no symptom response to proton pump inhibitors should be approached more cautiously by the surgeon. These patients may have another etiology for their symptoms, such as esophageal motility disorders, cardiac disease, pulmonary disease, or irritable bowel syndrome. The literature reports a symptom response to operative therapy of about 90%; although acid exposure decreases after the operation in almost all patients, it normalizes in about 80% of patients.

Textbook: Page 759 ANSWER: C

9. The following are true of complications of laparoscopic antireflux surgery except:

A. Pneumothorax caused by injury to the pleura during esophageal dissection is best treated with a chest tube.
B. Although dysphagia may be reported in up to 20% of patients, only 2% require dilation.
C. The most common cause of esophageal or gastric perforation during laparoscopic antireflux procedures is passage of the bougie.
D. Gastric perforation during a laparoscopic Nissen fundoplication is not an indication to convert to an open procedure.

DISCUSSION: Because the underlying lung is not injured and the CO_2 gas is rapidly absorbed from the pleural space, a chest tube is rarely needed to treat a pneumothorax. If the pleural defect can be closed, most of the gas is absorbed by the time the procedure is concluded. Supplemental oxygen is all that is necessary to treat a residual pneumothorax. Mild dysphagia is common immediately after an antireflux procedure; however, it usually abates after 1 to 2 months. It can be avoided by instructing the patient to adhere to a graduated viscosity diet during the 4 to 6 weeks after the operation. The most common cause of esophageal or gastric perforation is passage of the bougie. If the surgeon has the ability to repair the injury laparoscopically, then the procedure does not need to be converted to an open approach.

Textbook: Page 762 ANSWER: A

10. The following are true of paraesophageal hernias except:

A. They occur in the presence of a type II, III, or IV hiatal defect.
B. Anemia may be present in up to one third of patients.
C. The most common structure in the hernia sac is the stomach.
D. Gastric necrosis is common in patients with organoaxial volvulus.

DISCUSSION: Gastric necrosis is a rare complication in patients with paraesophageal hernias, even in the face of complete organoaxial volvulus. The reported rates range between 2 and 5%, and this is likely to be an overestimation since the true incidence of paraesophageal hernias is understated. Type II hiatal hernias are the pure rolling type of paraesophageal hernia in which the phrenoesophageal membrane keeps the gastroesophageal junction anchored in the abdomen. Type III hernias are a mixed sliding and rolling paraesophageal hernia, and type IV hernias involve an organ other than the stomach, which is the most commonly found structure in the hernia sac. Anemia may be found in over one third of patients due to the mucosal ischemia and bleeding that occurs.

Textbook: Page 767 ANSWER: D

11. Which of the following statements concerning the layers of the abdominal wall is correct?

A. Scarpa's fascia affords little strength in wound closure.

B. The internal abdominal oblique muscles have fibers that continue into the scrotum as cremasteric muscles.
C. The transversalis fascia is the most important layer of the abdominal wall in preventing hernias.
D. The lymphatics of the abdominal wall drain into the ipsilateral axillary lymph nodes above the umbilicus and into the ipsilateral superficial inguinal lymph nodes below the umbilicus.
E. All of the above.

DISCUSSION: The integrity of the abdominal wall is maintained by the transversalis fascia primarily. Scarpa's fascia affords little strength in wound closure, but its approximation aids considerably in the creation of an aesthetic scar. The cremasteric muscles of the spermatic cord are a continuation of muscle fibers from the internal abdominal oblique musculature. The lymphatic supply of the abdominal wall follows a simple pattern. These superficial lymphatics parallel the superficial veins, which above the umbilicus drain into the ipsilateral axillary vein and below the umbilicus drain into the ipsilateral femoral vein.

Textbook: Page 770 ANSWER: E

12. Which of the following congenital abnormalities is correctly defined?

A. Omphalocele represents a defect in the closure of the umbilical ring.
B. The herniated viscera associated with omphaloceles are usually covered with a membranous sac.
C. An umbilical polyp is a small excrescence of omphalomesenteric duct mucosa that is retained in the umbilicus.
D. Meckel's diverticulum results when the intestinal end of the omphalomesenteric duct persists and represents a true diverticulum.
E. All of the above.

DISCUSSION: Omphalocele may be seen in the newborn and represents a defect in the closure of the umbilical ring. The herniated viscera are usually covered with a sac. Gastroschisis is a defect of the abdominal wall lateral to the umbilical cord and is caused by failure of the closure of the body wall. The intestines protrude through the defect, and no sac is present to cover the herniated intestine. In the fetus, the omphalomesenteric duct may present as abnormalities related to the abdominal wall when the duct fails to obliterate. Meckel's diverticulum is the result of the failure of obliteration of the intestinal end of the omphalomesenteric duct. This is a true diverticulum with all layers of the intestinal wall represented. An umbilical polyp is a small excrescence of omphalomesenteric duct mucosa retained in the umbilicus. Such polyps resemble umbilical granulomas except they do not disappear after silver nitrate cauterization. Appropriate treatment is excision of the mucosal remnant.

Textbook: Page 774 ANSWER: E

13. Which of the following statements concerning desmoid tumors is correct?

A. These abdominal wall tumors are malignant fibrous tumors that arise from the musculoaponeurotic abdominal wall.
B. These tumors are histologically benign but frequently are locally invasive.
C. They usually present as a rapidly growing subcutaneous mass.
D. They have a high propensity toward metastasis.

DISCUSSION: Desmoid tumors of the abdominal wall are benign fibrous tumors that arise from the musculoaponeurotic abdominal wall. These tumors are histologically benign but frequently are locally invasive and are prone to recurrence following local excision. They present as firm, subcutaneous masses that grow slowly. They should be widely excised to prevent local recurrence. They do not have a propensity toward metastasis.

Textbook: Page 775 ANSWER: B

14. Which of the following statements is correct regarding retroperitoneal fibrosis?

A. Retroperitoneal fibrosis is relatively rare and about two thirds of all cases are considered idiopathic.
B. Presentation may vary from mild back pain to uremia or sepsis.
C. The characteristic findings are hydronephrosis and hydroureter proximal to the site of extrinsic compression of the ureters.
D. The ureters are generally deviated toward the midline.
E. All of the above.

DISCUSSION: Retroperitoneal fibrosis is a rare and unusual disease that has some similarities to hypersensitivity or autoimmune disease. The etiology is unknown and two thirds of all cases are considered idiopathic in that no specific cause can be proved. A correlation between the ingestion of methysergide and the disease has been reported. The most important clinical aspect of retroperitoneal fibrosis is that the fibrotic process frequently entraps and constricts the ureters, thereby causing obstructive uropathy. The patient's signs and symptoms depend on the presence or absence of urinary infection. The characteristic findings are hydronephrosis and hydroureters proximal to the site of extrinsic compression of the ureters. The disease is usually bilateral and results in deviation of the ureters toward the midline.

Textbook: Page 780 ANSWER: E

15. Which of the following statements concerning intraperitoneal fluid collections is correct?

A. Ascites occurs when either the peritoneal fluid secretion rate increases or the absorption rate decreases.
B. Accumulation of lymph within the peritoneal cavity usually results from trauma or tumor

involving the intra-abdominal lymphatic structures.
C. Choleperitoneum (intraperitoneal bile) generally occurs following biliary surgery, but spontaneous perforation of the bile duct has been reported.
D. The most common cause of hemoperitoneum is trauma to the liver or spleen.
E. All of the above.

DISCUSSION: Normally there is a balance between fluid secretion and absorption in the peritoneal cavity. Ascites occurs when either the secretion rate increases or the absorption rate decreases disproportionate to the other. Accumulation of lymph within the peritoneal cavity usually results from trauma or tumor involving lymphatic structures. Proposed treatment regimens range from salt restrictions and diuretics to surgical ligation and peritoneovenous shunting. Uninfected bile is a mild irritant to the peritoneal cavity and causes an increased production of peritoneal fluid, resulting in bile ascites or choleperitoneum. Most cases of choleperitoneum follow biliary tract surgery, but cases of spontaneous bile duct perforation have been reported in infants and some adults. The most common cause of hemoperitoneum is trauma to the liver or spleen. Less common causes include ruptured ectopic pregnancy, ruptured aortic aneurysms, or other intra-abdominal injuries.

Textbook: Page 776 ANSWER: E

16. The following statements about peritonitis are true except:

A. Peritonitis is defined as inflammation of the peritoneum.
B. Most surgical peritonitis is secondary to bacterial contamination.
C. Primary peritonitis has no documented source of contamination and occurs more commonly in adults than in children and occurs in men more than in women.
D. Tuberculous peritonitis can present with or without ascites.

DISCUSSION: Peritonitis is inflammation of the peritoneum and can be septic or aseptic, bacterial or viral, primary or secondary, acute or chronic. Most surgical peritonitis is secondary to bacterial contamination from the gastrointestinal tract. Primary peritonitis refers to inflammation of the peritoneal cavity without a documented source of contamination. It occurs more commonly in children than in adults and in women more than in men. This latter distribution is felt to be explained by entry of organism into the peritoneal cavity through the fallopian tubes. The clinical manifestations of tuberculous peritonitis are of two types. The moist form consists of fever, ascites, abdominal pain, and weakness. The dry form presents in a similar manner but without ascites.

Textbook: Page 777 ANSWER: C

17. Which of the following statements about cysts is not true?

A. Mesenteric cysts are most often due to congenital lymphatic spaces that gradually fill with lymph.
B. Mesenteric cysts usually present as abdominal masses accompanied by pain, nausea, or vomiting.
C. Mesenteric cysts are best treated by marsupialization.
D. Omental cysts are frequently asymptomatic unless they undergo torsion.

DISCUSSION: Mesenteric cysts are most often due to congenital lymphatic spaces that gradually enlarge as they fill with lymph. They generally present as abdominal masses accompanied by pain, nausea, and vomiting. They usually can be diagnosed on physical examination and have a characteristic lateral mobility. They are best treated by surgical excision, and intestinal resection may be necessary for their complete removal. Omental cysts are frequently asymptomatic but may present with vague discomfort or as a mobile abdominal mass that can cause torsion of the omentum. Torsion generally presents with signs and symptoms compatible with acute cholecystitis, appendicitis, or a twisted ovarian cyst. Treatment entails local resection.

Textbook: Page 779 ANSWER: C

18. What are the borders of the Hesselbach triangle?

A. Inferior epigastric vessels, rectus sheath, inguinal ligament.
B. Cooper ligament, lacunar ligament, rectus sheath.
C. Inguinal ligament, lacunar ligament, inferior epigastric vessels.
D. Cooper ligament, inferior epigastric vessels, femoral sheath.

DISCUSSION: The borders of Hesselbach triangle are (lateral) inferior epigastric vessels, (medial) rectus sheath, and (inferior) inguinal ligament.

Textbook: Page 784 ANSWER: A

19. The structure below which staples should not be placed during laparoscopic inguinal hernia repair is:

A. Medial iliopubic tract.
B. Cooper ligament.
C. Lateral iliopubic tract.
D. Inguinal ligament.

DISCUSSION: The structure below which staples should not be placed during laparoscopic inguinal hernia repair is the lateral (lateral to the internal inguinal ring) iliopubic tract.

Textbook: Page 792 ANSWER: C

20. The genitofemoral nerve root is:

A. L1–L2 or occasionally L3.
B. L1, L1–L2, or occasionally L3.
C. L2, L3.
D. T12, L1.

DISCUSSION: The genitofemoral nerve root is L1 or L1–L2, and occasionally L3.

Textbook: Page 785 ANSWER: B

21. Factors associated with hernia formation are:

A. Increase in hydroxyproline and abnormal proliferation of fibroblasts.
B. Increase in hydroxyproline and decrease in fibroblasts.
C. Decrease in hydroxyproline and decrease in fibroblasts.
D. Decrease in hydroxyproline and abnormal proliferation of fibrolasts.

DISCUSSION: Altered capacity for precipitation and reduced hydroxyproline ratio suggest impaired hydroxylation and lysyl oxidase activity. Synthesis of hydroxyproline results. Also, an abnormal proliferation of fibroblasts is seen in cells cultured from the rectus sheath of patients with groin hernias.

Textbook: Page 786 ANSWER: D

22. In the McVay repair:

A. Poupart ligament tendon is sutured to Cooper ligament from the pubic tubercle medially to the femoral canal.
B. The femoral canal is obliterated by a cone of mesh sutured to the surrounding structures with a nonabsorbable monofilament.
C. The conjoined tendon is sutured to Cooper ligament from the pubic tubercle laterally to the femoral canal.
D. Poupart ligament tendon is sutured to Cooper ligament from the pubic tubercle laterally to the femoral canal.

DISCUSSION: In the McVay (Cooper ligament) repair, the conjoined tendon is sutured to Cooper ligament from the pubic tubercle laterally to the femoral canal.

Textbook: Page 787 ANSWER: C

23. The safest time for abdominal surgery during pregnancy is:

A. First trimester.
B. Second trimester.
C. Third trimester.
D. Abdominal surgery is never safe during pregnancy.

DISCUSSION: Abdominal operations have been done throughout pregnancy with good outcomes. However, for elective or semielective procedures one should avoid operations during the first trimester to minimize fetal damage during the period of organogenesis. Also elective or semielective procedures should be done before the third trimester to avoid inducing premature labor.

Textbook: Page 813 ANSWER: B

24. The overall accuracy of computed tomography (CT) scanning in the diagnosis of acute appendicitis is:

A. 56%.
B. 27%.
C. 98%.
D. 77%.

DISCUSSION: Although CT scans can provide excellent accuracy in the diagnosis of acute appendicitis, one must remember that the data cited were obtained by expert radiologists using excellent equipment in a specialty center.

Textbook: Page 807 ANSWER: C

25. The diagnostic accuracy of laparoscopy in patients with acute abdominal pain is:

A. 24–30%.
B. 66–72%.
C. 93–100%.
D. 86–90%.

DISCUSSION: Laparoscopy can accurately reveal the cause of abdominal pain.

Textbook: Page 813 ANSWER: C

26. A 60-year-old man suddenly developed severe abdominal pain. In the emergency room 2 hours later his abdomen was soft and nontender, his white blood cell count was 18,300/mm^3, and his arterial blood pH was 7.32. The probable diagnosis is:

A. Acute appendicitis.
B. Acute pancreatitis.
C. Superior mesenteric artery embolism.
D. Perforated duodenal ulcer.

DISCUSSION: The sudden onset of severe abdominal pain, minimal or no physical findings, and marked leukocytosis point to acute visceral ischemia.

Textbook: Page 813 ANSWER: C

27. Which of the following is not a contraindication to laparoscopy in a patient with acute abdominal pain?

A. Hemodynamic instability.
B. Pregnancy.
C. Extensive abdominal distention.
D. History of multiple laparotomies.

DISCUSSION: Pregnancy was previously a contraindication to laparoscopy. However, clinical reports suggest that laparoscopy can be performed safely in pregnant patients.

Textbook: Page 813 ANSWER: B

28. A 39-year-old man presents with one episode of hematemesis 2 hours ago. He came immediately to the emergency room. He is hemodynamically stable and physical examination is normal. Endoscopy is performed that shows a clean-based shallow ulcer in the posterior wall of the first portion of the duodenum with mild associated antral gastritis. Which of the following is the most appropriate?

A. Endoscopic injection of sclerosing agent around the ulcer crater.
B. Biopsy of the gastric antrum for *Helicobacter pylori* testing.
C. Thermoprobe coagulation of the ulcer crater.

D. Admission to the intensive care unit (ICU) for 24 hours of monitoring.
E. Administration of sucralfate, 1 g PO q6h.

DISCUSSION: This 39-year-old man presents with an episode of hemorrhage from a bleeding duodenal ulcer without stigmata of hemorrhage. Therapeutic intervention is not appropriate for these clean-based shallow ulcers. ICU admission is not required for healthy young individuals. Rather, observation in a short-stay unit is appropriate. Optimal therapy includes use of an antisecretory agent, either an H_2-receptor antagonist, or a proton pump inhibitor. It is appropriate to biopsy the gastric antrum to determine if *H. pylori* is present. If performed, appropriate antibiotic treatment should be administered to eradicate this infection as well.

Textbook: Page 820 ANSWER: B

29. A 23-year-old woman presents with melena. Evaluation in the emergency room shows orthostatic hypotension, but physical examination is otherwise unremarkable. Upper endoscopy is normal. The most appropriate initial diagnostic test is:

A. Computed tomography scan of the abdomen.
B. Meckel scan.
C. Upper gastrointestinal and small bowel follow-through contrast study.
D. Mesenteric angiography.
E. Small bowel enteroscopy.

DISCUSSION: A 23-year-old patient with melena is most likely to have bleeding from Meckel's diverticulum. Additional sources to consider include bleeding from peptic ulceration in the gastroduodenal region. Emergency endoscopy is appropriate, as was completed in this case. Juvenile polyps and inflammatory bowel disease should also be included in the differential diagnosis. The most appropriate initial test after ruling out significant gastroduodenal ulceration is a Meckel scan. This test identifies approximately 70% of Meckel's diverticula, those that contain ectopic gastric mucosa. Acid secretion from the gastric mucosa induces ulceration of the adjacent small mucosa, leading to ulceration and hemorrhage. Colonoscopy would appropriately be completed after the Meckel scan in a patient of this age group if the Meckel scan is negative. Similarly, if the Meckel scan fails to diagnose a Meckel's diverticulum, upper gastrointestinal and small bowel follow-through would be appropriate for initial evaluation of the small bowel to identify Crohn's disease.

Textbook: Page 833 ANSWER: B

30. Dieulafoy's lesion of the gastric mucosa is characterized by:

A. Smooth submucosal mass with punctate central ulcerations.
B. Occult gastrointestinal blood loss.
C. Association with melanin spots on the lips.
D. An increased risk for gastric malignancy.
E. Episodic hemorrhage with no visible mucosal abnormalities on the gastric mucosa between episodes of hemorrhage.

DISCUSSION: Dieulafoy's lesions are large submucosal vascular abnormalities that bleed spontaneously. Hemorrhage is brisk and episodic. At endoscopy, no distinct mucosal abnormalities are noted unless the endoscopy is performed during a period of acute hemorrhage when brisk bleeding may be identified. The lesion is not associated with a risk for gastric malignancy, nor is melanin pigmentation of the lips, a characteristic of Peutz-Jeghers syndrome, noted. Submucosal masses with punctate ulceration are more characteristic of gastrointestinal stromal tumors or carcinoid.

Textbook: Page 828 ANSWER: E

31. Which of the following is true of acute gastric mucosal lesions?

A. Bleeding can usually be successfully controlled with arteriographic embolization.
B. They occur most commonly in patients with critical illness.
C. They are usually associated with epigastric pain.
D. Hemorrhage in these lesions carries a mortality rate of up to 10%.
E. They can be prevented with H_2-receptor antagonists at conventional doses.

DISCUSSION: Acute mucosal lesions occur in the setting of critical illness. Patients with elevated intracranial pressure, multisystem organ failure, coagulopathy, sepsis, and systemic inflammatory response syndrome are at greatest risk. These patients frequently have acid hypersecretion, particularly those with elevated intracranial pressure. Effective prophylaxis requires neutralization of gastric secretions. This may require dosing with an H_2-receptor antagonist at levels much higher than conventional dosing. These lesions are heralded by melanin, hematemesis, or coffee-ground material in nasogastric drainage secretions. Symptoms (e.g., abdominal pain) are rare. Hemorrhage from acute gastric mucosal lesions carries a high mortality. Persistent hemorrhage usually derives from multiple diffuse gastric mucosal erosions. Although arteriographic embolization may gain temporary control in 50 to 60% of patients, rebleeding is common unless the underlying medical predisposing risk factors are corrected. Persistent hemorrhage carries a mortality rate up to 50%.

Textbook: Page 827 ANSWER: B

32. It has been shown that *Helicobacter pylori* infection in the stomach is associated with each of the following except:

A. Chronic atrophic gastritis.
B. Gastric ulcer.
C. Duodenal ulcer.
D. Squamous cell carcinoma of the gastroesophageal junction.
E. Gastric adenocarcinoma.

DISCUSSION: Higher incidence of *H. pylori* infection has been reported in patients with chronic atrophic gastritis, gastric ulcer, duodenal ulcer, and gastric adenocarcinoma. There is no strong evidence to support the association of *H. pylori* infection and squamous cell carcinoma of the gastroesophageal junction.

Textbook: Page 845 ANSWER: D

33. Some patients following proximal gastric vagotomy or truncal vagotomy complain of "early satiety." The feeling of early satiety during meals is caused by:

A. Reduction in acid secretion following vagotomy.
B. Decreased force of gastric contraction.
C. Slow gastric emptying of liquids.
D. Slow gastric emptying of solids.
E. Loss of receptive relaxation of the fundus and upper body.

DISCUSSION: The stomach is normally collapsed when empty. The fundus relaxes during the deglutition process to start the process of accommodation as the stomach assumes its reservoir function. This "receptive relaxation" of the proximal stomach is mediated through vagal inhibitory reflexes. Proximal gastric, or truncal, vagotomy interferes with this receptive relaxation so that the arrival of the ingested food to the stomach is associated with a relatively high increase in intragastric pressure. The increase in intragastric pressure accounts for the feeling of early satiety described by some patients following vagotomy. None of the other answers are the causes of early satiety following the procedure.

Textbook: Page 840 ANSWER: E

34. Which one of the following statements most accurately reflects current understanding of the pathophysiology of peptic ulcer disease?

A. Most patients with *Helicobacter pylori* infection develop peptic ulcer disease.
B. Hypersecretion of acid alone is the cause of duodenal ulcer but not of gastric ulcer disease in over 50% of the patients.
C. Acid plays a role as a cofactor in *H. pylori* or peptic ulcer disease associated with nonsteroidal anti-inflammatory drugs (NSAIDs).
D. Gastric acid plays a very minor or no role in the development of peptic ulcer disease.
E. Gastritis is rarely noted in patients with gastric ulcer disease.

DISCUSSION: Although most patients with peptic ulcer disease are infected by *H. pylori,* most patients with *H. pylori* infection do not progress to peptic ulcer disease. The yearly incidence of peptic ulcer in *H. pylori*–infected adults is only about 1%. Hypersecretion of acid alone rarely is the cause of duodenal or gastric ulcer with the exception of Zollinger-Ellison syndrome and idiopathic hypersecretory disorders. However, acid plays an important role as a cofactor in *H. pylori* or NSAIDs-associated peptic ulcer disease. Antral gastritis is frequently noted in patients with gastric ulcer, particularly those who are also infected with *H. pylori*.

Textbook: Page 844 ANSWER: C

35. Elevated serum gastrin is found in all of the following conditions except:

A. Retained antrum.
B. Gastric outlet obstruction.
C. Postvagotomy.
D. Duodenal ulcer associated with *Helicobacter pylori* infection.
E. Pernicious anemia.

DISCUSSION: It has been well documented in clinical studies that serum gastrin level is elevated in postvagotomy patients and patients with retained antrum and pernicious anemia. The mechanism for elevated gastrin in these patients is largely due to the high pH of gastric contents. Gastrin production is inhibited by low pH of the gastric juice as part of the feedback mechanism. Gastric outlet obstruction causes elevated gastrin level because of gastric distention, which is one of the stimulatory factors for gastrin production. Duodenal ulcer associated with *H. pylori* has not been shown to cause hypergastrinemia.

Textbook: Page 654 ANSWER: D

36. All of the following statements concerning gastric cancer are correct except:

A. Both the incidence and the mortality of gastric cancer increase with age.
B. The incidence and mortality of gastric cancer have progressively declined during the last half-century in low-incidence but not in high-incidence areas throughout the world.
C. The declining incidence of gastric cancer has been due to a decrease in the incidence of the intestinal subtype in both high- and low-risk populations, whereas the diffuse subtype has been increasing in most low-risk populations.
D. Gastric cancer occurs more frequently in men.

DISCUSSION: The incidence and mortality of gastric cancer have progressively declined during the last half-century in both low- and high-incidence areas throughout the world.

Textbook: Page 856 ANSWER: B

37. All of the following have been reported to increase the risk of gastric cancer except:

A. Cigarette smoking.
B. *Helicobacter pylori* infection.
C. Alcohol consumption.
D. Previous gastric resection.
E. Chronic atrophic gastritis.

DISCUSSION: Alcohol consumption does not increase the relative risk for gastric cancer.

Textbook: Page 857 ANSWER: C

38. All of the following statements about the treatment of gastric cancer are true except:

A. Selection of the proper surgical procedure to effect a curative resection is determined primarily by the location of the primary tumor within the stomach and the need to obtain margins around the tumor of at least 5 cm.
B. Total gastrectomy that is unnecessary to obtain adequate gastric wall margins does not improve patient survival.
C. Prophylactic splenectomy does not improve survival for similarly staged patients with gastric cancer.
D. Patients with gastric cancer should routinely receive adjuvant chemotherapy following resection.
E. Five-year survival following resection of early gastric cancer varies between 70 and 95% depending on whether lymph node metastases are present or not.

DISCUSSION: Although encouraging data have been reported from Japan where adjuvant chemotherapy is considered standard and is initiated immediately during the postoperative period or even intraoperatively, adjuvant chemotherapy following curative resection has not been demonstrated to be of value in Western countries with the regimens tested to date. Presently, adjuvant chemotherapy for gastric cancer cannot be recommended outside of carefully controlled clinical trials.

Textbook: Pages 862–865 ANSWER: D

39. All of the following are true concerning gastric lymphoma except:

A. Primary gastric lymphoma most commonly involves the fundus of the stomach.
B. Most mucosa-associated lymphoid tissue–derived gastric lymphomas are of B-cell origin and derive from a distinct lineage of B cells.
C. Primary gastric lymphomas are curable by complete surgical resection alone.
D. Radiotherapy and chemotherapy, alone or in combination, result in survival rates comparable to those achieved with surgical treatments.
E. Primary gastric lymphoma is not associated with bone marrow or peripheral lymph node involvement and has a pattern of metastasis similar to that of gastric cancer.

DISCUSSION: Primary gastric lymphoma most commonly involves the antrum, followed by the body and then the cardia, although it can extend to involve the entire stomach.

Textbook: Page 865 ANSWER: A

40. In contrast to ulcerative colitis, Crohn's disease of the colon:

A. Is not associated with increased risk of colon cancer.
B. Frequently presents with daily hematochezia.
C. Is usually segmental rather than continuous.
D. Has a lower incidence of perianal fistulas.
E. Never develops toxic megacolon.

DISCUSSION: Crohn's disease of the colon is a patchy, segmental, chronic, transmural inflammatory process that penetrates the bowel wall to form fistulas but seldom causes rectal bleeding. In contrast, ulcerative colitis is a mucosal ulcerating process that extends continuously from the rectum to the more proximal colon and frequently results in bleeding. In both diseases toxic megacolon can develop, and both predispose the patient to increased risk of malignancy of the large intestine over the long term.

Textbook: Page 889 ANSWER: C

41. Options to consider when operating for Crohn's disease of the large intestine include all of the following except:

A. Colectomy and ileoproctostomy.
B. Colectomy, closure of the rectal stump, and ileostomy.
C. Segmental colectomy with colocolonic anastomosis.
D. Proctocolectomy and Brooke ileostomy.
E. Proctocolectomy and ileoanal J pouch.

DISCUSSION: Patients with colonic Crohn's disease who have minimal or mild rectal involvement can be treated by segmental colectomy with colocolonic anastomosis; colectomy and ileoproctostomy; or colectomy, closure of the rectal stump, and ileostomy. When severe rectal involvement is also present, proctocolectomy with permanent ileostomy is required. The ileoanal pouch procedure is not performed for Crohn's disease because of the risk of recurrence of Crohn's disease in the ileal pouch in the postoperative period.

Textbook: Page 895 ANSWER: E

42. Crohn's disease:

A. Is caused by mumps virus.
B. Is more common in Asians than in Jews.
C. Tends to occur in families.
D. Is less frequent in temperate climates than in tropical ones.
E. Is improved by smoking.

DISCUSSION: The cause of Crohn's disease is unknown. No specific microorganism has been identified as a pathogen, and no clear-cut environmental factor, such as smoking, has been implicated, even though many patients with Crohn's disease are heavy smokers. The disease does tend to occur in families. It is more common among Jews than Asians and among people who live in temperate climates than those in tropical ones.

Textbook: Page 888 ANSWER: C

43. Recurrence after operation for Crohn's disease:

A. Occurs after operations for ileal Crohn's but not colonic Crohn's.

B. Is usually found just proximal to an enteric anastomosis.
C. Rarely requires reoperation.
D. Occurs in 1% of patients at risk per year during the first 10 years after the operation.
E. Is prevented by maintenance therapy with corticosteroids.

DISCUSSION: Recurrence after operation for Crohn's disease often occurs just proximal to an enteric anastomosis or stoma and occurs at a rate of about 6% per year over the first 10 years after operation. Recurrence follows operations for both ileal and colonic Crohn's and is not prevented by medical therapy using corticosteroids. Reoperation is required for 30 to 50% of subjects at risk.

Textbook: Page 895 ANSWER: B

44. Excision rather than bypass is preferred for surgical treatment of small intestinal Crohn's disease because:

A. Excision is safer.
B. Bypass does not relieve symptoms.
C. Excision cures the patient of Crohn's disease but bypass does not.
D. Fewer early complications appear with excision.
E. The risk of small intestine cancer is reduced.

DISCUSSION: Bypass of segments of small bowel affected with Crohn's disease is a safe operation with few complications, and one that usually relieves symptoms promptly. It leaves diseased bowel behind, however, which can flare in the future and develop carcinoma. Excision, although it does not cure Crohn's disease, removes the areas of severe involvement and so eliminates the risk of developing cancer in these segments.

Textbook: Pages 893–895 ANSWER: E

45. Cholecystokinin (CCK) is believed to function in all of the following processes except:

A. Delays gastric emptying.
B. Plays a role in satiety regulation.
C. Contracts the gallbladder.
D. Stimulates pancreatic secretion.
E. Controls the anal sphincter.

DISCUSSION: CCK has a physiologic role in the regulation of gastric emptying, eating behavior, gallbladder contraction, and pancreatic secretion. There is experimental evidence that it may serve as a neurotransmitter in the function of the lower esophageal sphincter. It probably also has a role in augmenting the release of insulin after a meal. It has no known role in the function of the anal sphincter.

Textbook: Page 880 ANSWER: E

46. All of the following statements about the embryology of Meckel's diverticulum are true except:

A. Meckel's diverticulum usually arises from the ileum within 90 cm of the ileocecal valve.
B. Meckel's diverticulum results from the failure of the vitelline duct to obliterate.
C. The incidence of Meckel's diverticulum in the general population is 5%.
D. Meckel's diverticulum is a true diverticulum encompassing all layers of the intestinal wall.
E. Gastric mucosa is the most common ectopic tissue found within a Meckel's diverticulum.

DISCUSSION: Meckel's diverticulum is a true diverticulum containing all layers of the intestinal wall, usually arising from the antimesenteric border of the ileum 45 to 90 cm proximal to the ileocecal valve. It is a vestige of the omphalomesenteric or vitelline duct, which usually undergoes complete obliteration during the seventh week of gestation. Autopsy studies have estimated the incidence of Meckel's diverticulum to be 1 to 2%, with men being more commonly affected than women by a ratio of 2:1. Gastric mucosa is present in 50% of all Meckel's diverticula, but is seen in over 75% of symptomatic individuals.

Textbook: Page 907 ANSWER: C

47. Which statement about carbohydrate digestion is false?

A. Amylopectin has 1,4 straight chains and 1,6 side chains.
B. Amylase breaks 1,4 glucose linkages.
C. Amylase breaks 1,6 side chains.
D. An adult may ingest about 350 g of carbohydrate daily.
E. Dietary starch contains two glucose polymers, amylopectin and amylase.

DISCUSSION: Amylopectin, the most abundant constituent of starch, is a 1,4-linked straight chain of glucose molecules. In addition, amylopectin possesses a 1,6 branching side chain at approximately every 25 glucose units along the straight chain. Pancreatic and salivary amylase break the interior 1,4 glucose linkages.

Textbook: Page 876 ANSWER: C

48. Extensive resection of the small bowel, leaving only 2 or 3 feet beyond the ligament of Treitz anastomosed to the transverse colon, can lead to the following metabolic complications except:

A. Gastric hyperacidity and hypersecretion.
B. Hyperoxaluria.
C. Hypermetabolic response.
D. Fat-soluble vitamin deficiency.
E. Cholelithiasis.

DISCUSSION: Once the stress of the surgical procedure is over, there is no further hypermetabolic response, nor does there appear to be any reduced energy expenditure from loss of the metabolically active small bowel. Energy needs are unaltered. Gastric secretion and hyperacidity are directly related to the extent of small bowel resection and are due in part to increased concentrations of gastrin in the serum. H_2-blockers are effective in reducing acidity and volume of gastric secretions. Hyperoxaluria develops due to binding of calcium to fat in the diet with steatorrhea, leaving less calcium to bind with dietary oxalate. The soluble oxalate is absorbed by the colon and excreted in the urine. If oxalate is excessive, oxalate kidney stones can form. With fat malabsorption due to bile salt depletion and rapid intestinal transit, absorption of the fat-soluble vitamins A, E, K, and D is reduced. Even with oral supplementation, deficiencies can develop.

Textbook: Page 912 ANSWER: C

49. Which of the following physical factors of irradiation is related to the potential for radiation injury?

A. The dimension of the radiation portals.
B. The number of portals.
C. The number of fractions.
D. The total amount of irradiation.
E. All of the above.

DISCUSSION: These physical factors are interactive. Less energy is delivered through a small portal than through a large one. Multiple portals permit concentration of the radiation in the area to be treated and spare skin and viscera from damage. There is less risk of injury from irradiation of a given intensity if more fractions are applied.

Textbook: Page 911 ANSWER: E

50. All of the following describe effects and uses of the hormone somatostatin except:

A. Inhibition of gastrin release.
B. Stimulation of pancreatic secretion.
C. Symptomatic treatment for carcinoid syndrome.
D. Useful in the symptomatic treatment of esophageal variceal bleeding.
E. Inhibition of intestinal secretion.

DISCUSSION: Somatostatin is considered the universal off-switch that inhibits the release of many hormones as well as inhibiting pancreatic and gastric secretion and intestinal motility. The clinical uses of somatostatin include treatment of intestinal fistulas, most notably pancreatic fistulas; the treatment of hormone-overproducing endocrine tumors; and symptomatic treatment of esophageal variceal bleeding.

Textbook: Page 880 ANSWER: B

51. A 35-year-old man with Crohn's disease has had two prior bowel resections, including an ileocolectomy, for complications related to Crohn's disease. He has approximately 100 cm of small bowel remaining and is currently readmitted for a high-grade bowel obstruction that has not responded to conservative measures. At laparotomy, three strictures are noted over a length of 50 cm. The management should be:

A. Three separate segmental bowel resections with primary anastomoses.
B. Resection of the 50-cm segment of involved small bowel with reanastomosis.
C. Insertion of a long intestinal tube extending past the most distal stricture.
D. Three stricturoplasties.
E. A bypass of the strictured segment by a side-to-side jejunocolic anastomosis.

DISCUSSION: The guiding principle in the surgical management of Crohn's disease is to resect a portion of bowel specifically involved in the complicated process. Repeated wide resections result in no greater remissions or cure, and can lead to the devastating short bowel syndrome. Therefore, resection of the 50-cm segment of involved small bowel would not be prudent given the prior resections. Bypass is infrequently used. Insertion of a long intestinal tube would be a short-term solution; however, it would not alleviate the problem. The best option in this patient with previous intestinal resections would be to perform stricturoplasties that effectively widen the lumen but avoid resection.

Textbook: Pages 893–894 ANSWER: D

52. Of the following, the best treatment for symptoms related to the superior mesenteric artery syndrome is:

A. Gastrojejunostomy with vagotomy.
B. Resection of the superior mesenteric artery and placement of a polytetrafluoroethylene graft.
C. Duodenojejunostomy.
D. Pancreaticoduodenectomy.
E. Total parenteral nutrition.

DISCUSSION: Treatment of patients with superior mesentery artery syndrome varies. Conservative measures are tried initially and have been increasingly successful as definitive treatment. If surgery is required, the treatment of choice is duodenojejunostomy.

Textbook: Page 913 ANSWER: C

53. Which of the following statements about jejunoileal diverticula is not true?

A. These are classified as true diverticula.
B. Patients may present with chronic abdominal pain.
C. The majority of the diverticula are located on the mesenteric side.
D. The blind loop syndrome may be associated with these diverticula.
E. Jejunoileal diverticulosis is an acquired abnormality.

DISCUSSION: The great majority of patients with jejunoileal diverticula remain asymptomatic. However, patients may present with chronic symptomatology including vague, chronic abdominal pain; malabsorption; and chronic low-grade gastrointestinal hemorrhage. Diverticula of the small bowel are false diverticula that protrude on the mesenteric side of the intestine. The etiology of jejunoileal diverticulosis is thought to be motor dysfunction of the smooth muscle or the myenteric plexus resulting in discoric contractions of the small bowel. Other complications of this disease include diverticulitis, hemorrhage, intestinal obstruction, and blind loop syndrome. Jejunoileal diverticulosis is an acquired abnormality and not congenital.

Textbook: Page 903 ANSWER: A

54. A patient with a strangulating obstruction of the small bowel may be differentiated from a simple obstruction by:

A. Fever.
B. Leukocytosis.
C. Elevated levels of serum D-lactate.
D. Elevated ammonia levels.
E. None of the above.

DISCUSSION: Classic signs of a strangulating obstruction have been described and include tachycardia, fever, leukocytosis, and a constant noncramping abdominal pain. However, a number of studies have conclusively shown that no clinical parameters or laboratory measurements can accurately detect or exclude the presence of strangulation in all cases. Various serum determinations have been evaluated including lactate and ammonia levels; however, to date, no single laboratory examination can accurately predict strangulating obstruction.

Textbook: Page 886 ANSWER: E

55. Which of the following statements regarding Crohn's disease and cancer of the small bowel and colon is true?

A. Cancers of the small bowel typically occur in the duodenum.
B. In general, the prognosis is better in Crohn's patients with colon cancer compared with patients with colon cancer not associated with Crohn's disease.
C. The frequency of cancer is similar in patients with extensive, long-standing Crohn's colitis and those with extensive ulcerative colitis.
D. Chemotherapy is more effective in the treatment of metastatic lesions arising from colonic cancers in patients with Crohn's disease.
E. The occurrence of cancer is not related to the duration and extent of Crohn's colitis.

DISCUSSION: Long-standing Crohn's disease predisposes to cancer of both the small intestine and colon. The relative risk for adenocarcinoma of the small bowel and Crohn's disease is at least 100-fold greater than in matched controls. Although this relative risk of small bowel cancer and Crohn's disease is quite high, the absolute risk is still small. Of greater concern is the development of colorectal cancer in patients with colonic involvement and a long duration of disease. Recent evidence indicates that with the same duration and anatomic extent of disease, the risk of cancer and Crohn's disease of the colon is as great as with ulcerative colitis. Most cancers associated with Crohn's disease are not detected until in the advanced stages and prognosis is generally poor.

Textbook: Pages 891, 895 ANSWER: C

56. The most common malignant neoplasm of the small bowel is:

A. Primary adenocarcinoma.
B. Lymphoma.
C. Leiomyosarcoma.
D. Metastatic neoplasm.
E. Carcinoid tumor.

DISCUSSION: Of the primary malignant neoplasms of the small bowel, adenocarcinoma and carcinoid tumors are the most common neoplasms depending on the series examined. However, metastatic tumors involving the small bowel are much more common than primary neoplasms. Small intestinal involvement is either by direct extension or implantation of tumor cells, although metastasis from extra-abdominal tumors may also be found, particularly with adenocarcinoma of the breast, carcinoma of the lung, and melanoma.

Textbook: Page 899 ANSWER: D

57. Which of the following statements about duodenal diverticula is true?

A. Duodenal diverticula are relatively uncommon.
B. The majority of duodenal diverticula are located in the third and fourth portions of the duodenum.
C. If found incidentally during laparotomy for another condition, diverticula of the duodenum should be resected if this is easily accomplished.
D. Over 50% of patients with duodenal diverticula experience a major complication at some point during their lifetime.
E. Complications of duodenal diverticula include cholangitis, hemorrhage, and perforation.

DISCUSSION: Diverticula of the duodenum are relatively common, representing the second most common site for diverticulum formation after the colon. The typical location of duodenal diverticula is in the second portion of the duodenum; however, approximately 10% of duodenal diverticula develop more distally and laterally. Diverticula can be found in the periampullary region projecting from the medial wall of the duodenum. The important thing to remember is that the overwhelming majority of duodenal diverticula are asymptomatic and are usually noted incidentally. Less than 5% of duodenal diverticula require operation because of a complication of the diverticulum itself. Major complications of duodenal diverticula include obstruction of the biliary or pancreatic ducts that may contribute to cholangitis and pancreatitis, hemorrhage, perforation and, rarely, blind loop syndrome. If found incidentally during laparotomy for another condition, these diverticula should be left alone.

Textbook: Page 905 ANSWER: E

58. Which of the following statements about the surgical treatment of carcinoid tumors is false?

A. Carcinoid tumors should be treated by resection, regardless of the presence of metastases.
B. Appendiceal tumors greater than 1.5 cm should be treated by ileocolectomy.
C. Local excision with margins is adequate for a rectal carcinoid of any size.
D. Carcinoid tumors are associated with a large percentage of other synchronous or metachronous neoplasms.
E. In the gastrointestinal tract, carcinoid tumors of the appendix and small bowel are the most common.

DISCUSSION: Carcinoid tumors should be treated by resection, regardless of the presence of metastases, because growth of the primary neoplasm is slow and local complications, such as obstruction and intussusception, are frequent. At clinical discovery, a large percentage (as many as 70%) of small intestinal carcinoids are metastatic to lymph nodes and/or liver. All tumors should be managed by wide en bloc resection, regardless of the size of the primary lesion or the presence of distant metastases. Lesions in the distal ileum require ileocolectomy. Appendiceal tumors >1.5 cm should be treated by ileocolectomy. The incidence of metastases depends on the size and location of the primary tumor. Appendiceal carcinoid tumors <1.5 cm are rarely malignant and may be treated safely by routine appendectomy. This is not true of larger tumors. Like carcinoid tumors elsewhere in the gastrointestinal tract, the malignancy potential of rectal carcinoid tumors is directly proportional to their size. Tumors <1 cm have little or no malignant potential and may be treated by endoscopic excision. Tumors measuring 1 to 2 cm should be excised operatively with margins, but when tumors are >2 cm, rectal carcinoid tumors may require anterior resection. In patients with ileal carcinoid tumors, the incidence of a second tumor has been reported as high as 40%. Thus, the search for synchronous metachronous and metastatic neoplasms should be undertaken.

Textbook: Pages 903–904, 994 ANSWER: C

59. Which of the following statements about carcinoid syndrome are true?

A. Carcinoid syndrome occurs only when hepatic metastases are present.
B. Serotonin is thought to be responsible for the diarrhea, cardiac lesions, and flushing in patients with carcinoid syndrome.
C. Foregut carcinoid tumors cause atypical carcinoid syndrome; hindgut tumors are rarely, if ever, associated with the syndrome.
D. The long-acting somatostatin analogue is predominantly effective in inhibiting tumor growth but has minimal effects on the symptoms associated with the carcinoid syndrome.
E. Carcinoid tumors and the carcinoid syndrome are commonly associated with multiple endocrine neoplasia (MEN) Type 2A.

DISCUSSION: Carcinoid syndrome occurs when venous drainage from the tumor gains access to the systemic circulation, escaping hepatic degradation. Although hepatic metastases are most often responsible, retroperitoneal metastases and bronchial, ovarian, and testicular carcinoid tumors can also cause the carcinoid syndrome. Serotonin is thought to be largely responsible for both the diarrhea and the fibrosing cardiac lesions associated with the carcinoid syndrome. The vasomotor changes, however, are mediated by kinins and vasoactive peptides such as substance P, neuropeptide K, neurokinin A, and neurotensin. Other substances, such as histamine, vasoactive intestinal peptide (VIP) and prostaglandins, may also contribute to systemic manifestations in the carcinoid syndrome. Foregut carcinoid tumors, of which stomach and bronchial tumors are the most common, can cause atypical carcinoid syndrome. It is thought that these tumors are deficient in the enzyme dopa-decarboxylase and have impaired conversion of 5-hydroxytryptophan (5-HTP) into 5-hydroxytryptamine (5-HT), leading to secretion of 5-HTP into the vascular compartment. Some of the 5-HTP is converted into 5-HT and 5-hydroxyindoleacetic acid (5-HIAA) in extrarenal sites, and some is decarboxylated in the kidney and excreted into the urine as 5-HT; but some of the 5-HTP is excreted directly into the urine. Thus, in patients with foregut tumors, the urine contains relatively little 5-HIAA (but more than normal) but large amounts of 5-HTP and 5-HT, in contrast to patients with midgut carcinoid tumors, in whom large amounts of 5-HIAA are secreted into the urine but relatively little 5-HTP. Carcinoid tumors of the hindgut contain no argentaffin or argyrophil cells, they have no secretory products, and therefore they are not associated with the carcinoid syndrome. The long-acting somatostatin analogue provides the best symptomatic therapy because somatostatin inhibits both release and action of humoral mediators of the carcinoid syndrome. By contrast, serotonin antagonists are of little value, and the efficacy of interferon therapy has yet to be established.

Textbook: Pages 901–904 ANSWER: C

60. Correct treatment for a 2-cm appendiceal carcinoid at the base of the appendix is:

A. Appendectomy with inversion.
B. Subtotal abdominal colectomy.
C. Right hemicolectomy with ileocolostomy.
D. Colostomy with mucous fistula.
E. None of the above.

DISCUSSION: The correct treatment for a large appendiceal carcinoid at the base of the appendix is right hemicolectomy with primary anastomosis because the chance of metastases to the liver as well as the regional lymph nodes is higher with larger tumors. In addition, since it is at the base of the appendix, there may be residual tumor left if a simple appendectomy is done. Appendectomy with inversion would leave residual tumor and subtotal abdominal colectomy is more than is necessary, as is colostomy with mucous fistulas. Therefore, the safest procedure to remove all disease while limiting morbidity is a right hemicolectomy and ileocolostomy.

Textbook: Page 918 ANSWER: C

61. The most common complication of acute appendicitis is:

A. Intra-abdominal abscess.
B. Bowel obstruction secondary to adhesions.
C. Pneumonia.
D. Wound infection.
E. None of the above.

DISCUSSION: In general, most patients with acute, nonperforated appendicitis do well. These patients are usually young and have a short hospital stay. However, active appendiceal inflammation does increase the risk of a local wound infection. In most patients, however, the overall risk with nonperforated appendicitis is under 5%.

Textbook: Page 925 ANSWER: D

62. Incidental appendectomy is probably of most benefit in which of the following surgical procedures?

A. Nephrectomy for Wilms' tumor.
B. Cholecystectomy.
C. Hysterectomy.
D. Cystectomy.
E. Exploration for Crohn's disease of the terminal ileum.

DISCUSSION: Incidental appendectomy has been done in conjunction with all of the procedures listed; however, the incidence of complications is frequently increased when an incidental appendectomy is done with these procedures. This is particularly true for certain operations such as nephrectomy for Wilms' tumor. Since recurrent bouts of Crohn's disease of the terminal ileum can be mistaken for appendicitis, when Crohn's disease of the terminal ileum is found at exploration for possible appendicitis, an appendectomy should be performed in order to prevent misdiagnosis in the future. Although some investigators have been worried that appendectomy in the face of Crohn's disease may increase the risk of fistula formation, this has generally not proved to be an issue if good closure of the appendiceal stump is achieved.

Textbook: Page 918 ANSWER: E

63. Most patients with acute, nonperforated appendicitis will:

A. Culture multiple bacteria from the peritoneal cavity.
B. Demonstrate a fecalith on plain abdominal radiographs.
C. Require short-term (<24 hours) antibiotic treatment.
D. Be hospitalized for 5 to 7 days.

DISCUSSION: Antibiotics are given as prophylaxis to patients with nonperforated appendicitis. Because the peritonitis is very localized and of short duration, these patients do not need a lengthy course of therapy and a single perioperative dose of the appropriate agent or agents almost always suffices. This is in contradistinction to patients with perforated appendicitis in whom the peritonitis is already established. These patients need several days or longer of antibiotic treatment.

Textbook: Page 922 ANSWER: C

64. The most common bacteria found in patients with perforated appendicitis is:

A. *Bacteroides fragilis.*
B. *Staphylococcus aureus.*
C. *Pseudomonas aeruginosa.*
D. *Klebsiella pneumoniae.*

DISCUSSION: The *Bacteroides fragilis* group of bacteria are the most common anaerobic bacteria found in patients with perforated appendicitis. Numerous bacteriologic studies over the past 60 years have documented this. *Bacteroides* are not the most common bacteria present in fecal culture, but they do have a greater pathogenic potential than some of the other enteric anaerobes. It is thought that the capsule present in *B. fragilis* is an important virulence factor.

Textbook: Page 919 ANSWER: A

65. The appendix is:

A. Derived from the forgut.
B. Usually found in a retrocecal location.
C. Supplied by a branch of the inferior mesenteric artery.
D. Located along the path of the gubernacular descent.

DISCUSSION: There is occasionally some confusion about the normal location of the appendix. The appendix is found just posterior to the cecum in about 60% of patients; hence it is most commonly retrocecal. This should not be confused with the retroperitoneal, retrocecal location, which is an infrequent (<2%) occurrence. The end of the cecum is normally an intraperitoneal structure.

Textbook: Page 917 ANSWER: B

66. Criteria for a sonographic diagnosis of appendicitis include all of the following except:

A. Appendicolith.
B. Noncompressible appendix.
C. Appendiceal diameter greater than 7 mm.
D. Inflamed psoas muscle.

DISCUSSION: Sonographic diagnosis of appendicitis depends on visualization of the appendix, and typically a noncompressible appendix of greater than 7 mm diameter is diagnostic for appendicitis. An appendicolith is also diagnostic for appendicitis. Although an inflamed psoas muscle is a nonspecific sign of inflammation in the right lower quadrant, it cannot be used specifically for the diagnosis of appendicitis.

Textbook: Page 921 ANSWER: D

67. (True or False) Barium enema is a useful technique to diagnose appendicitis.

A. True.
B. False.

DISCUSSION: Barium enema is not typically a useful technique to diagnose appendicitis. There are a number of problems with this technique. Most specifically, incomplete filling of the tip of the appendix can yield a false-negative study. Nonspecific signs of indentation of the cecum are used as markers of inflammation in the right lower quadrant and are notoriously unreliable. Barium enema also hampers the use of computed tomography and ultrasonography for future imaging investigations.

Textbook: Page 921 ANSWER: B

68. The optimal initial treatment for patients with a preoperatively diagnosed appendiceal mass includes:

A. Laparoscopic appendectomy.
B. Intravenous antibiotics alone.
C. Percutaneous drainage and antibiotics.
D. Open appendectomy.

DISCUSSION: The optimal treatment for patients with a preoperatively diagnosed appendiceal mass is percutaneous drainage and antibiotics if indeed this is a periappendiceal abscess. If this is a phlegmon, then intravenous antibiotics alone could potentially be used, but this is somewhat controversial. Laparoscopic appendectomy or open appendectomy are not typically used as the initial treatment in patients who have a clearly identified perforated or complex appendicitis with periappendiceal abscess formation.

Textbook: Page 924 ANSWER: C

69. The motility pattern of the gastrointestinal (GI) tract is:

A. Constant throughout the gastrointestinal tract.
B. Variable with propulsive retropulsive waves throughout the GI tract.
C. Characterized by only propulsive waves throughout the colon.
D. Consists of propulsive waves throughout the GI tract except in the right colon where there is also retropulsive waves.

DISCUSSION: Regarding motility, the right colon is the exception of all segments of the human GI tract because its normal pattern includes retropulsive waves. The purpose of these waves is to create stasis and allow fermentation by anaerobic bacteria.

Textbook: Page 934 ANSWER: D

70. Regarding colonic function, which of the following statements is true?

A. The right colon is the main site of bacterial fermentation.
B. The left colon is the main site of storage of feces.
C. The rectum is the main site of fluid and electrolyte absorption.
D. Because life expectancy is not changed following total colectomy, there is no discernible function for the colon.

DISCUSSION: In terms of function, the colon can be divided into three units: the right colon, the left colon, and the rectum. The right colon is the main site for bacterial fermentation, the left colon is the site for water and electrolyte absorption, and the rectum is the main site for storage of feces. Although life expectancy is not changed following total colectomy, there are some sequelae from the loss of colonic function such as a predisposition to nephrolithiasis (dehydration) and gallstones (interruption of bilioenteric circulation of bile salts).

Textbook: Page 934 ANSWER: A

71. When imaging the colon for diagnosing intrinsic pathology.

A. Computed tomography (CT) scan is highly sensitive for cancer surveillance.
B. Barium enema is helpful in staging rectal cancer.
C. Defecography demonstrates the various forms of colonic dysmotility.
D. Abdominal ultrasonography is safe and effective in acute diverticulitis.

DISCUSSION: CT scan is helpful in staging colorectal cancer, but to date has not been useful for cancer surveillance. However, virtual colonoscopy is a new modality that can be generated by CT scanning and promises a high degree of resolution allowing for cancer surveillance. Colonic transit time studies, and not defecography, are helpful in diagnosing colonic dysmotility. Abdominal ultrasound is very helpful, and very safe, in patients with diverticulitis. A diverticular abscess can be demonstrated by ultrasound, and a drainage catheter can be placed in the abscess using ultrasound for guidance.

Textbook: Page 937 ANSWER: D

72. Regarding endoscopic examination of the colon and rectum:

A. The main advantage of endoscopy over imaging is that it allows for biopsies.
B. The flexibility of the colonoscope makes its use safe in acute diverticulitis.
C. The advantage of rigid over flexible sigmoidoscopy is that it does not require bowel preparation.
D. Endoscopy is highly helpful in toxic megacolon.

DISCUSSION: There is no form of endoscopy that is safe in acute diverticulitis. Endoscopy requires insufflation of air which can break the seal over a perforated diverticulum and create diffuse peritonitis or directly perforate the wall in cases of toxic megacolon. Both forms of endoscopy, rigid and flexible, require bowel preparation. However, endoscopy is very helpful in establishing tissue diagnosis by biopsy of colonic lesions.
Textbook: Page 936 ANSWER: A

73. Bowel preparation prior to colonic surgery:

A. Improves healing of colonic anastomoses.
B. Reduces the likelihood of leakage of colonic anastomoses.
C. Minimizes the morbidity of dehiscence of colonic anastomoses.
D. Overcomes the impairment in healing created by the use of corticosteroids.

DISCUSSION: Although there are some reports questioning the benefits of bowel preparation, most surgeons operating on the colon agree that bowel preparation minimizes the morbidity of dehiscence of colonic anastomoses. However, eliminating fecal bulk does not necessarily create better conditions for healing. In fact, the colon derives nutrients from its luminal contents in the form of short-chain fatty acids (SCFA). SCFA are produced by bacteria and their production is drastically reduced by bowel preparation. Therefore, bowel preparation does not favor colonic healing.
Textbook: Page 940 ANSWER: C

74. The use of laparoscopic techniques in colonic surgery:

A. Reduces postoperative discomfort.
B. Reduces operating time.
C. Extends the long-term survival of patients with colorectal cancer.
D. Reduces the cost of surgery.

DISCUSSION: Laparoscopy in colorectal surgery is still in evolution. Although it does reduce postoperative discomfort, it does not reduce operating time or cost. There is significant concern of disseminating cancer cells through the use of pneumoperitoneum. Therefore, many surgeons would consider cancer a contraindication for laparoscopic resection.
Textbook: Page 967 ANSWER: A

75. An erect abdominal x-ray of cecal volvulus typically includes all of the following features except:

A. Air-fluid levels throughout the small bowel.
B. Paucity of air in the small bowel.
C. A "bird's beak" sign in the right lower quadrant.
D. Large air-fluid level in the left upper quadrant.

DISCUSSION: A cecal volvulus produces a distal small bowel obstruction; therefore, the finding of air-fluid levels in the small bowel is quite typical. The "bird's beak" sign usually points to where the torsion occurred (right lower quadrant), while the cecum and ascending colon turn up into the left lower quadrant.
Textbook: Page 947 ANSWER: B

76. Treatment options for patients with sigmoid volvulus include all of the following except:

A. Preoperative endoscopic reduction and stenting with large-bore tube.
B. Preoperative fluid resuscitation and prophylactic antibiotics.
C. Sigmoid resection, end-colostomy, and closure of the rectum (Hartmann procedure).
D. Operative reduction and replacement of sigmoid colon along the left paracolic gutter.

DISCUSSION: Patients with sigmoid volvulus are usually elderly and debilitated, and their colons are irreversibly dilated and aperistaltic. Therefore, simple reduction is never a good option for these patients. All other options are appropriate and very helpful.
Textbook: Pages 948–950 ANSWER: D

77. All of the following are organs that can be affected in patients with ulcerative colitis except:

A. Colon.
B. Duodenum.
C. Liver.
D. Eyes.

DISCUSSION: Patients with ulcerative colitis have inflammatory changes limited to the colon. However, extraintestinal manifestations can involve the liver (i.e., sclerosing cholangitis) and eyes (i.e., uveitis). The duodenum is not affected by ulcerative colitis.
Textbook: Page 950 ANSWER: B

78. All of the following types of polyps carry a risk of malignant transformation except:

A. Tubulous.
B. Villous.
C. Tubulovillous.
D. Juvenile.

DISCUSSION: Villous adenomas carry the higher risk of malignant transformation. However, tubular and tubulovillous adenomas are also premalignant neoplasias. Juvenile (hypertrophic) polyps do not seem to have malignant potential.
Textbook: Page 958 ANSWER: D

79. The hereditary nonpolyposis colorectal cancer syndromes are transmitted via:

A. The proto-oncogene *K-ras*.
B. The tumor suppressor gene *APC*.
C. Mismatch repair genes.
D. The risk modifier gene *CD44v*.

DISCUSSION: Different forms of colorectal cancer can now be linked to specific genetic derangements. The hereditary nonpolyposis colorectal cancer syndromes are associated with defects in the mismatch repair genes such as the *hMSH2* and *MLH1*.

Textbook: Page 956 ANSWER: C

80. In patients with hereditary nonpolyposis colorectal cancer.

A. Colon cancer typically presents in the left side.
B. Women with the Type I form can also have ovarian cancer.
C. The typical age of presentation is in the early 40s.
D. Cancers are more aggressive than the sporadic type of the same cancer.

DISCUSSION: In patients with hereditary nonpolyposis colorectal cancer syndromes the typical age of presentation is in the early 40s. As opposed to sporadic types, cancer usually presents in the right side of the colon and tends to be less aggressive. The Type II form is associated with endometrial cancer and cancers of the urinary epithelium.

Textbook: Page 961 ANSWER: C

81. Typical presentations of patients with colorectal cancer include:

A. Early obstructive symptoms in right colon tumors.
B. Chronic anemia in left colon tumors.
C. Bleeding and mucus discharge in rectal tumors.
D. Palpable mass in splenic flexure tumors.

DISCUSSION: Typically, tumors in the right colon produce chronic anemia whereas tumors of the left colon produce obstruction. Tumors in the transverse colon, and particularly in the splenic flexure, are usually asymptomatic until they produce either obstruction or perforation. The typical presentation of rectal tumors is bleeding and mucus discharge which are often attributed to hemorrhoids.

Textbook: Page 965 ANSWER: C

82. All of the following are forms of therapy with proven efficacy in colorectal cancer except:

A. Preoperative radiation in rectal tumors.
B. Surgery alone in cecal tumors.
C. Chemotherapy alone in sigmoid tumors.
D. Surgery alone in transverse colon tumors.

DISCUSSION: Preoperative radiation has been proved to be beneficial in rectal tumors whereas surgery is the treatment of choice in all forms of colorectal cancer. Chemotherapy has not been proved of benefit in colorectal cancer.

Textbook: Pages 966–967 ANSWER: C

83. Which of the following statements is true concerning the maintenance of continence?

A. It depends on both the internal and external sphincters as well as the puborectalis.
B. Resting pressure offers a high-pressure zone that increases resistance to the passage of stools.
C. Maximal squeeze pressure can last no more than 1 minute.
D. All of the above.

DISCUSSION: Continence depends on numerous complex and interrelated anal, rectal, pelvic floor, and colonic factors. Resting pressure depends primarily on the internal sphincter and serves to increase resistance to the passage of stool. Squeeze pressure, generated by contraction of the external sphincter, increases anal canal resting pressure and helps prevent leakage when the rectal content is presented to the proximal anal canal at inopportune times. It lasts but a minute before fatiguing. The anorectal angle produced by the anterior pull of the puborectalis encircles the rectum at the level of the anorectal ring and also aids in continence.

Textbook: Page 975 ANSWER: D

84. Which of the following statements is true about complete rectal prolapse or procidentia?

A. Rectal prolapse results from an intussusception of the rectum and rectosigmoid.
B. The disorder is more common in men than in women.
C. Continence nearly always recovers after correction of the prolapse.
D. All of the above.

DISCUSSION: Rectal prolapse is believed to be the result of intussusception of the rectum and rectosigmoid. The condition predominates in women, in those who strain excessively, and in those suffering from mental disorders. Pregnancy and delivery are not implicated, as the condition can be observed in men and in nulliparous women. By the time the diagnosis is secured, 50% of patients are incontinent and continence improves in only half of the patients after surgical correction of the prolapse.

Textbook: Page 978 ANSWER: A

85. Which of the following statements regarding hemorrhoids is not true?

A. Hemorrhoids are specialized "cushions" present in everyone to aid continence.
B. External hemorrhoids are covered by skin, while internal hemorrhoids are lined by mucosa.
C. Pain is often associated with uncomplicated hemorrhoids.
D. Hemorrhoidectomy is reserved for third- and fourth-degree hemorrhoids.

DISCUSSION: Hemorrhoids are specialized, highly vascularized cushions present in the anal canal to aid continence. The cause of hemorrhoids is unknown, but they may be no more than the downward sliding of anal cushions associated with straining and irregular bowel habits. They are classified and treated according to the degree of their symptoms. External hemorrhoids are covered with anoderm and are distal to the dentate line. Internal hemorrhoids are covered by the mucosal lining of the anal canal proximal to the dentate line. They can cause painless bleeding, usually associated with defecation. Pain is usually not associated with uncomplicated hemorrhoids but more often occurs with fissures. Hemorrhoidectomy is reserved for third-degree (bleeding with prolapse requiring manual reduction) and fourth-degree (permanently prolapsed with or without bleeding) hemorrhoids.

Textbook: Page 979 ANSWER: C

86. The widely accepted treatment of most localized epidermoid, cloacogenic, or transitional cell carcinoma of the anal canal is:

A. Abdominoperineal resection.
B. Chemotherapy alone.
C. Radiotherapy alone.
D. Combination of chemoradiation.

DISCUSSION: Tumors arising in the anal canal or in the transitional zone that have squamous, basaloid, cloacogenic, or mucoepidermoid epithelium share a similar behavior in clinical presentation and response to treatment. Combined chemoradiation, or so-called Nigro protocol, promises to preserve continence, avoid colostomy, and offer similar survivorship. Local excision is reserved for the few, very small and superficial lesions. For most lesions, chemoradiation including external beam radiation, 5-fluorouracil, and mitomycin C is the primary treatment of choice.

Textbook: Page 992 ANSWER: D

87. Which of the following statements is true with regard to hidradenitis suppurativa?

A. It is a disease of the apocrine sweat glands.
B. It causes multiple perianal and perineal sinuses that drain watery pus.
C. The sinuses do not communicate with the dentate line.
D. The treatment is surgical.
E. All of the above.

DISCUSSION: Hidradenitis suppurativa is an inflammatory process of the sweat glands characterized by abscess and sinus formation. The disease may involve other areas where apocrine glands are present such as the axilla, mammary, inguinal, and genital regions. The affected areas have a blotchy, purplish appearance with numerous sinuses draining watery pus. The condition must be differentiated from cryptoglandular fistulas, which communicate with the dentate line and Crohn's disease, which may tract to the anorectum proximal to the dentate line. Treatment consists of unroofing sinuses in limited disease and wide local excision in more advanced disease.

Textbook: Page 989 ANSWER: E

88. All of the following are true regarding acute anal fissures except:

A. They produce pain and bleeding with defecation.
B. Women typically have anterior fissures.
C. They result from sphincter hypertonia and mucosal ischemia.
D. They can be treated successfully with nitric oxide.

DISCUSSION: Anal fissures are linear ulcers that occur in the distal anal canal. Although women are more likely to have an anterior fissure than men, both men and women are more likely to have a posterior midline fissure. If the fissure is chronic, it is typically associated with a sentinel pile and a hypertrophied anal papilla. Fissures can usually be diagnosed by inspecting the anal verge, although at times they may require anoscopy or examination under anesthesia for patients who have a deep buttock or are difficult to examine owing to hypertonia. First-line therapy typically includes sitz baths, bran, or bulking agents. If there is no relief with these simple measures, the fissures should then be treated with "reversible chemical sphincterotomy" with nitroglycerin or isosorbide-dinitrate or, that failing, they can be treated with partial lateral internal sphincterotomy. "Medical" and surgical sphincterotomy are thought to work by relieving anal hypertonia and mucosal ischemia.

Textbook: Page 981 ANSWER: B

89. Anorectal abscesses are infections that typically:

A. Originate within anal crypt glands.
B. Resolve completely without sequelae after incision and drainage.
C. Form horseshoe extensions.
D. Occur in patients who are immunocompromised.
E. Can be treated early with antibiotics.

DISCUSSION: By far the vast majority of anorectal abscesses are of cryptoglandular origin rather than from Crohn's disease or hidradenitis suppurativa. Crypt infections spread in the intersphincter plane giving rise most often to ischiorectal or perianal abscesses and infrequently giving rise to horseshoe extensions. Antibiotics may delay the diagnosis of deep abscess but do not provide definitive treatment. Abscesses occur in healthy patients and in immunocompromised patients, the latter of whom require more aggressive management to avoid systemic sepsis. Although incision and drainage may be the final episode of treatment for some patients, many will go on to form a fistula from the primary opening to the incision drainage site. For that reason it is best to perform the incision and drainage outside the region of the sphincter, to avoid damage, but otherwise as close to the anus as possible. This should allow for a shorter track for any subsequent fistulotomy.

Textbook: Page 983 ANSWER: A

90. Regarding fistula in ano:

A. The majority are intersphincteric.
B. They usually follow a curvilinear course to the midline if arising in the anterior anal crypts.

C. Persistent drainage after fistulotomy indicates the presence of Crohn's disease.
D. Seton placement should rarely be required.

DISCUSSION: Fistulas represent the long-term sequelae of anorectal abscesses. The most common types are the intersphincteric and transphincteric, with suprasphincteric and extrasphincteric fistulas, fortunately, being quite rare. To avoid false tracks at the time of fistulotomy, it is best to start the examination of the fistula track by probing inside the anal canal at the level of the dentate line. Following Goodsall rules—that is, anterior fistulas track in a direct line radial from the secondary to the primary opening, and posterior fistulas track curvilinear to the midline—the primary offending crypt can usually be identified. Fistulas are best managed by direct fistulotomy when minimal sphincter muscle is involved, by delayed fistulotomy with a seton for anterior fistulas in women and for fistulas with extensive sphincter involvement, and with sphincter-preserving techniques such as fibrin glue injection and local advancement flaps in more complex fistulas that involve all or nearly all of the sphincter muscle. Incomplete division of the track or management of a high blind end can lead to persistent symptoms after fistulotomy. On rare occasions, persistence of a fistula track may indicate the presence of Crohn's disease, but this is rare in the absence of other gastrointestinal manifestations of Crohn's.

Textbook: Page 985 ANSWER: A

91. All of the following are true regarding rectovaginal fistulas except:

A. Etiologies include congenital and acquired conditions.
B. They are often diagnosed based on symptoms alone.
C. For a high rectovaginal fistula, rectal resection is almost always necessary.
D. Successful repair of a low rectovaginal fistula requires maximal resolution of inflammatory diseases.

DISCUSSION: Rectovaginal fistulas may be congenital or acquired; those that are acquired are most often due to trauma, typically obstetrical or surgical. Rectovaginal fistulas are best described as being high or low within the vagina, as this greatly influences the surgical approach. Fistulas that are high within the vagina require a transabdominal approach with or without rectal resection according to the nature and extent of the underlying rectal involvement. Correction may require little more than dissection and interposition of a pedicle of tissue such as omentum, or it may require, in fact, a very extended operation such as low anterior resection or coloanal anastomosis. Low fistulas are best managed once the acute period of inflammation has resolved (usually 3 to 6 months). These can be treated with a number of approaches including transvaginal, transrectal, transperineal, transsphincteric, and transanal procedures. The fistula can be completely excised and the complete perineal laceration repaired in layers, or it can be closed with a sliding advancement flap, which is less often successful but is less disruptive to the sphincter muscles.

Textbook: Page 986 ANSWER: C

92. Which statement is true of patients with Crohn's disease who present with an anorectal problem?

A. They usually require proctectomy.
B. They are best managed conservatively.
C. The anal condition is always related to the Crohn's process.
D. They should not be considered for sphincterotomy.

DISCUSSION: Patients with Crohn's disease may present with anal manifestations including fissures, fistulas, and abscesses. Anal manifestations may become extensive and severe enough to necessitate proctectomy but this is uncommon. In assessing the patient with the possibility of Crohn's of the perineum, one should evaluate the remainder of the gastrointestinal tract to establish the extent of active disease. Patients with Crohn's disease may have common disorders of the anus such as fissures and hemorrhoids, or they may have true manifestations of perineal Crohn's disease. The characteristic appearance of Crohn's includes edematous purplish tags, and deep wide-based fissures with granulation tissue. Fistulas typically have large incompletely drained cavities and typically arise above the level of the dentate line, as opposed to cryptoglandular disease which originates at the level of the dentate line. Surgery is indicated for Crohn's of the perineum to ensure complete drainage of infection with or without the use of a seton. Treatment with metronidazole and immunosuppressive agents is indicated. For those patients who have Crohn's disease and common anal conditions such as fissures and cryptoglandular abscesses and fistulas, these conditions can be treated using standard approaches; however, caution is advised against aggressive approaches especially when there is uncertainty as to the true nature of the disease.

Textbook: Page 990 ANSWER: C

93. Wide local excision is least likely to be indicated in which of the following?

A. Bowen's disease.
B. Paget's disease.
C. Squamous cell carcinoma of the anal margin.
D. Squamous cell carcinoma of the anal canal.
E. Basal cell carcinoma of the anus.

DISCUSSION: It is of paramount importance to differentiate anal canal from anal margin lesions. Anal margin tumors are most often treated as skin tumors, that is, little more than wide local excision and close follow-up are required. This is certainly true for squamous cell carcinoma of the anal margin and basal cell carcinoma of the anus. Although squamous cell carcinoma of the anal canal can be treated with wide local excision when it presents in a very early stage, most often these tumors are treated with combined radiation-chemotherapy. In situ squamous cell carcinoma (Bowen's disease) and in situ adenocarcinoma (Paget's disease) are also amenable to wide local excision assuming there is no underlying invasive component. Paget's disease is more likely to have an underlying component and an aggressive multimodality approach for these invasive tumors is more appropriate. For Paget's disease and Bowen's disease, in which the extent of the tumor is often difficult to discern on visual inspection alone, it is essential to perform mapping procedures using histology to determine the extent of the tumor and establish negative tumor margins.

Textbook: Page 994 ANSWER: D

94. Verrucous carcinomas are:

A. Often fast-growing.
B. Always invasive.
C. Rarely known to metastasize.
D. Essentially the same as squamous cell carcinomas.

DISCUSSION: Verrucous carcinomas are tumors with an aggressive potential that is somewhere intermediate between condyloma acuminatum and invasive squamous cell carcinoma. They typically present as large warty lesions that are slow-growing. They can present with local complications including fistula, infection, or even malignant degeneration. Radical wide local excision is appropriate for noninvasive lesions, but abdominoperineal resection is advised for lesions that cannot be controlled with local excision or that have an invasive component.

Textbook: Page 992 ANSWER: C

95. For melanoma of the anal canal, the following are true except:

A. They are often amelanotic.
B. Abdominoperineal resection is the procedure of choice.
C. Five-year survival rates are poor at 10 to 17%.
D. Survival rates are stage-dependent.

DISCUSSION: Melanomas involving the anal canal are not infrequently amelanotic at the time of presentation. Because these tumors are quite rare, it is difficult to draw hard and fast conclusions; however, it appears the 5-year survival rate is more dependent on stage of disease than on the procedure performed. Whether results from abdominoperineal resection are superior to those from local excision remains debated, even though it has been reported that 5-year survivors are typically those undergoing abdominoperineal resection for early lesions. Regardless of the procedure performed, the overall 5-year survival rate is very poor, around 10 to 17%. There is no apparent role for prophylactic inguinal node dissection.

Textbook: Page 994 ANSWER: B

NOTES

NOTES

NOTES

NOTES

CHAPTER 12

LIVER, BILIARY, SPLEEN, PANCREAS

1. The common bile duct receives a rich supply of blood from which of the following vessels?

A. Anterior and posterior communicating branches from the pancreatic artery.
B. Medial and lateral segmental branches from the hepatic artery.
C. Superior and inferior branches from the gastric artery.
D. Three o'clock and 9 o'clock vessels from the gastroduodenal and hepatic arteries.
E. Twelve o'clock and 6 o'clock vessels from the gastroduodenal and hepatic arteries.

DISCUSSION: The blood supply of the common bile duct arises from the gastroduodenal, common hepatic, and right hepatic arteries. A plexus formed on the duct provides two axial vessels, the 3 o'clock and 9 o'clock arteries, named for their positions relative to a cross section of the duct.

Textbook: Page 1003 ANSWER: D

2. In Rappaport's description of the hepatic lobule, Zone 3 is closest to which of the following vessels?

A. Portal venules.
B. Hepatic arterioles.
C. Central hepatic veins.
D. Lymph vessels.
E. None of the above.

DISCUSSION: The hepatocytes around the portal venule are divided arbitrarily into three zones. Zone 1 is the area immediately adjacent to the portal venule, where the sinusoids are smaller in diameter with many collaterals. Zones 2 and 3 are farther away from the portal venule, and Zone 3 is closest to the central vein of the acinus.

Textbook: Page 1004 ANSWER: C

3. The triangle of Calot is bounded by which of the following structures?

A. Cystic duct, common hepatic duct, liver.
B. Gallbladder, common bile duct, portal veins.
C. Right hepatic duct, left hepatic duct, liver.
D. Portal vein, right hepatic artery, liver.
E. Pancreatic neck, liver, duodenum.

DISCUSSION: The triangle bounded by the cystic duct, common hepatic duct, and the hilum of the liver is the triangle of Calot. Detection of this anatomic triangle is useful during cholecystectomy because the cystic artery passes through these borders.

Textbook: Page 1004 ANSWER: A

4. Lack of urobilinogen in the urine is most commonly associated with which of the following conditions?

A. Complete biliary obstruction.
B. Ethanol-induced pancreatitis.
C. Overgrowth of intestinal bacteria.
D. Diarrhea.

DISCUSSION: Part of urobilinogen is resorbed in the intestine and excreted in the urine. With complete biliary obstruction, urobilinogen cannot form and, therefore, does not appear in the urine. Ethanol-induced pancreatitis, overgrowth of intestinal bacteria, and diarrhea do not interfere with urobilinogen secretion by the liver.

Textbook: Page 1009 ANSWER: A

5. What is the term for the regeneration of glucose from lactate by the liver?

A. Krebs cycle.
B. Anaerobic metabolism.
C. Cori cycle.
D. Aerobic metabolism.
E. None of the above.

DISCUSSION: Lactate produced by anaerobic metabolism is metabolized only in the liver. Ordinarily it is converted to pyruvate and subsequently back to glucose. This shuttling of glucose and lactate between liver and peripheral tissue is carried out in the Cori cycle. The Krebs cycle involves degradation of the 2-carbon acetyl group of acetyl coenzyme A producing ATP, a process that occurs in most tissues. Aerobic and anaerobic metabolism are energy-producing processes that use or do not use oxygen, respectively.

Textbook: Page 1009 ANSWER: C

6. Which of the following procoagulant factors is not synthesized in the liver?

A. Fibrinogen.

B. Factor VII.
C. Von Willebrand's factor.
D. Factor IV.
E. Factor X.

DISCUSSION: The liver synthesizes 11 proteins critical for hemostasis, which include all the procoagulant factors except von Willebrand's factor. This procoagulant is a large, multimeric protein that circulates in the blood plasma and is stored in endothelial cells and platelets. Von Willebrand's factor is secreted from platelets and endothelial cells in response to appropriate stimuli.
Textbook: Page 1010 ANSWER: C

7. All of the following are correct regarding sinusoidal blood flow except:
A. The sinusoids empty into terminal hepatic venules that drain into the hepatic veins.
B. The sinusoids are the major site for the regulation of blood flow, hepatic capacitance, and solute exchange.
C. Hepatic sinusoids are 7- to 15-μm wide with very low resistance (2 to 3 mm Hg).
D. The hepatic artery supplies most of the blood to the sinusoids.
E. Sinusoidal membranes are highly permeable.

DISCUSSION: Most blood enters the sinusoids from the portal venules guarded by inlet sphincters. Hepatic artery blood predominantly supplies the biliary system, including intrahepatic and extrahepatic bile ducts. A minimal amount of arterial blood enters the sinusoids directly through sinoarterial twigs.
Textbook: Page 1006 ANSWER: D

8. Which of the following statements regarding laparoscopic staging of hepatobiliary cancer is incorrect?
A. Laparoscopic ultrasound is a useful adjunct to laparoscopic staging in hepatobiliary surgery.
B. Laparoscopy and laparoscopic ultrasound allow for the assessment of resectability in hepatobiliary malignancies.
C. Tumor size and lymph node involvement but not the degree of cirrhosis can be estimated with laparoscopic staging and laparoscopic-guided biopsy.
D. Other radiologic imaging studies can be replaced by laparoscopic staging in hepatobiliary malignancies.
E. Laparoscopic staging can be performed immediately preceding laparotomy.

DISCUSSION: Laparoscopy enables surgeons to detect and biopsy small lesions not only in the liver but also on the peritoneum or diaphragm. Additionally, an assessment of the entire liver can be made at the time of laparoscopy, and the severity of cirrhosis assessed with laparoscopically guided biopsy. Sensitivity rates for the detection of satellite lesions in hepatobilary cancer with intraoperative ultrasound have approached 90 to 100%.
Textbook: Page 1035 ANSWER: C

9. All of the following regarding hemobilia are true except:
A. The venous system is more commonly involved than the arterial system due to the increased incidence of aneurysmal rupture.
B. It may be caused by trauma (iatrogenic/accidental), tumor, infection, or pressure necrosis.
C. The gold standard and most commonly employed diagnostic modality is angiography.
D. The classic triad of symptoms and signs includes gastrointestinal bleeding, jaundice, and right upper quadrant pain.
E. Although helpful in diagnosis and treatment in a significant percentage of cases, endoscopic retrograde cholangiopancreatograpy (ERCP) or percutaneous transhepatic cholangiography (PTC) can confuse the diagnosis by causing new sources of bleeding.

DISCUSSION: The arterial system is most commonly involved due to the higher pressure in this system. Iatrogenic trauma has become a more important cause over the past few decades due to the increasing array of diagnostic and therapeutic techniques involving the hepatobiliary region. The other choices have been classically described to cause hemobilia. Angiography is the most sensitive test to isolate the bleeding source. Therapeutic management by coiling or other embolization techniques can be performed using this modality. Statement D is the classic triad put forth by Sandblom. There is approximately a two-thirds incidence for each component of the triad. Trauma caused by ERCP and PTC can cause difficulty in isolating the original bleeding site in some cases. These modalities are also commonly implicated as causes of de novo hemobilia when employed for other reasons.
Textbook: Page 1056 ANSWER: A

10. Which of the following statements is true concerning the management of echinococcal disease of the liver?
A. Because of the risk of rupture, pericystectomy is not recommended.
B. The recurrence rate following ablation is similar to that following resection.
C. Hypertonic saline, formalin, 80% alcohol, and 0.5% cetrimide are commonly used as scolecidal agents in ablation.
D. Sclerosing agents should be used following all ablation procedures to minimize recurrence.
E. Following ablation, drainage is accompanied by greater postoperative morbidity and prolonged hospitalization than by obliteration alone.

DISCUSSION: Except in cases with biliary communication, the drainage of echinococcal cysts following ablation is accompanied by greater postoperative morbidity and prolonged hospitalization. Therefore, most surgeons prefer not to drain the cyst cavities. Many surgeons still practice ablation despite its higher recurrence rate. Hypertonic saline, chlorhexidine, 80% alcohol, and 0.5% cetrimide are all useful as scolecidal agents and may be instilled into the cyst cavity. Because of the potential for biliary tract injury, a sclerosing solution should not be used when the cyst communicates with the biliary system.

Textbook: Page 1055 ANSWER: E

11. Which of the following statements is true regarding hepatic amebiasis?

A. The infection is most commonly transmitted by person-to-person contact rather than by contaminated food and water.
B. An increasing incidence is seen among homosexual men.
C. Active disease is present when trophozoites or cysts are found in the stool.
D. The abscesses tend to rupture intraperitoneally when found in the left lobe.
E. Diagnosis is usually made by aspirating protozoans from abscesses.

DISCUSSION: The most common mode of transmission of *Entamoeba histolytica* is by individual contact. Although the prevalence of amebiasis in homosexual men is higher than the rest of the population on average (20 to 30%), this prevalence is dropping secondary to decreased high-risk behavior. The presence of trophozoites or cysts in the stool in itself does not confirm the presence of active disease. Although 75 to 90% of amebic abscesses are found in the right lobe, resulting in a higher number of intraperitoneal ruptures in general, those abscesses that occur in the left lobe more commonly rupture into the pericardial or pleural spaces. Because *E. histolytica* organisms are found only in a rim of necrotic tissue, they are unlikely to be found in abscess aspirates.

Textbook: Page 1048 ANSWER: A

12. Which of the following statements is true in the management of pyogenic abscess?

A. Untreated abscesses are fatal in 50 to 75% of cases.
B. Drainage should be performed as soon as the diagnosis is made in all cases of pyogenic abscess.
C. Drainage procedures have obviated the need for hepatic resection.
D. Percutaneous drainage with antibiotics is the preferred method of treatment, with success rates approaching 90%.
E. Follow-up imaging is required in all cases of image-guided drainage catheter placement.

DISCUSSION: Percutaneous drainage with antibiotics is successful in treating pyogenic abscess in 85 to 90% of cases, and because of its low morbidity has become the treatment of choice. Untreated abscesses are 95 to 100% fatal, primarily due to rupture with subsequent sepsis. An initial 1- to 2-day period of intravenous antibiotics, especially in cases of multiple abscesses, is often beneficial prior to drainage. Abscesses secondary to hepatic malignancy and chronic granulomatous disease of childhood are unlikely to respond to drainage and antibiotics. As a result, liver resection is indicated in these patients. Only those patients who fail to improve clinically following image-guided drainage catheter placement should have follow-up computed tomography or ultrasound.

Textbook: Page 1050 ANSWER: D

13. Which of the following statements is correct in the management of amebic abscess?

A. Those cases without bacterial superinfection have a posttreatment mortality rate of 20 to 30%.
B. The treatment of choice includes initial drainage with metronidazole.
C. The usual duration of metronidazole treatment is 4 to 6 weeks.
D. Most cases of ruptured abscess involve the chest.
E. Surgical drainage is generally reserved for right lobe abscesses.

DISCUSSION: Of those cases of amebic abscess that rupture, 10 to 20% are intrathoracic, 2 to 7% are intra-abdominal, and 2% are intrapericardial. The mortality from drained abscesses in the absence of bacterial superinfection should be less than 5%. Most uncomplicated cases respond to 7 to 14 days of metronidazole treatment without drainage. Surgical drainage, although rare, is reserved for large left-lobe amebic abscesses not amenable to percutaneous drainage following failed medical management.

Textbook: Page 1052 ANSWER: D

14. Which of the following statements is true in regard to hepatocellular carcinoma (HCC)?

A. It is decreasing in incidence in the United States.
B. It is shifting to an older population in the United States.
C. It occurs more commonly in men due to genetic predisposition.
D. It has doubled in the United States since the 1970s.
E. It is among the 10 most common primary malignancies in the United States.

DISCUSSION: Five different studies demonstrate HCC to have doubled since the 1970s in the United States. The overall incidence of HCC in the United States has increased from 1.4 per 100,000 during the period of 1976 to 1980 to 2.4 per 100,000 from 1991 to 1995. Although increasing age is associated with a higher risk for HCC, recent data suggest that incidence in the United States is shifting to a slightly younger demographic (40 to 60 years old) than previously noted. The higher risk for men in certain populations probably reflects a greater exposure to environmental carcinogens. The differences include not only a higher hepatitis B carrier rate in males but also dietary carcinogens and varying rates of metabolism between the sexes. HCC makes up a relatively small proportion of the total primary cancers diagnosed on a yearly basis in the United States. It has an annual incidence in the United States of 1 to 7 per 100,000 population and is the twenty-second most common type of cancer.

Textbook: Page 1020 ANSWER: D

15. Which of the following statements is true in the detection of hepatocellular carcinoma (HCC)?

A. Approximately 25% of patients present with signs and symptoms of metastatic lesions, of which the lungs are the most common site.
B. Hepatomegaly is the most common sign at presentation.
C. Increased carcinoembryonic antigen (CEA) is found in 20 to 30% of patients.
D. Alpha-Fetoprotein (AFP) is more sensitive in detection than des-gamma-carboxy-prothrombin (DGCP) as a marker for lesions of all sizes.
E. Obstructive jaundice is the initial sign in 20 to 30% of patients.

DISCUSSION: Hepatomegaly is the most common sign at presentation. Approximately 5% of patients present with a manifestation of metastatic lesions, of which pulmonary metastases are the most common. Increased CEA occurs in 8% of cases. DGCP has a sensitivity of 70% and a specificity of 100%, superior to AFP only in tumors more than 5 cm in size. Obstructive jaundice is the initial problem in 1 to 10% of patients.

Textbook: Page 1022 ANSWER: B

16. Which of the following statements is true regarding the diagnostic modalities used for hepatocellular carcinoma (HCC)?

A. Computed tomography (CT) is not sensitive for lesions smaller than 1 cm.
B. Transabdominal ultrasonography and radionuclide scans are not sensitive in detecting lesions smaller than 1 to 2 cm.
B. Preoperative laparoscopy has a limited role in the diagnosis of HCC.
C. Percutaneous biopsy is necessary in directing the surgical management of these patients.
D. Hepatic arteriography offers no benefit in the management of these patients.

DISCUSSION: Transabdominal ultrasonography and radionuclide scans are not sensitive in detecting lesions smaller than 1 to 2 cm. A recent study of the literature demonstrated that CT is highly sensitive at detecting HCC, even when the lesions are smaller than 1 cm (sensitivity 95 to 96%). Laparoscopy is emerging as a procedure of choice in the diagnosis of HCC or other suspected liver tumors. Five separate studies demonstrated its usefulness before anticipated resection, particularly in the detection of occult metastases not demonstrated by other modalities. Laparoscopy also offers an opportunity for limited treatment. Percutaneous needle biopsy or fine-needle aspiration for cytodiagnosis generally adds little to the evaluation of potentially resectable, indeterminate liver masses; in addition, needle biopsy or aspiration has some hazard for hypervascular masses. Hepatic arteriography is occasionally helpful in determining the extent of the disease and, in particular, portal or arterial involvement. It can also predict the usefulness of direct arterial infusion or chemoembolization for HCC, which may be hypervascular or hypovascular. A preoperative arteriogram may also be helpful in determining anatomic variability. A distinct disadvantage of arteriography is the possibility of thrombosing an artery to the remaining lobe when major hepatic resection is anticipated.

Textbook: Page 1022 ANSWER: B

17. Which of the following is true concerning the pathology of hepatocellular carcinoma (HCC)?

A. The fibrolamellar variant of HCC occurs more commonly in younger females and has a more favorable prognosis than standard HCC.
B. The fibrolamellar variant accounts for 10 to 20% of HCC, and occurs most commonly in the right lobe.
C. Carcinosarcoma is more commonly metastatic than standard HCC and has a worse prognosis.
D. The clear cell carcinoma variant is often confused with metastatic clear cell lung cancer.
E. Childhood HCC is most commonly unilateral and unifocal.

DISCUSSION: The fibrolamellar variant of HCC occurs more commonly in younger patients and has a more favorable prognosis than standard HCC. The neoplasm includes only 1 to 2% of all HCCs, but it accounts for as many as 40% of such tumors in patients younger than 35 years old. A female sex predilection is debated. Two thirds of such tumors occur in the left lobe. Although carcinosarcoma metastases may be more common than standard HCC, these patients may actually live longer than those with the more common HCC. Clear cell HCC is often difficult to distinguish from metastatic renal cell carcinoma. In fact, the two tumors have been found to coexist in the same patients. In most cases, the gross features of childhood HCC include multifocality and bilaterality.

Textbook: Page 1024 ANSWER: A

18. Which statement is true regarding survival in patients with hepatocellular carcinoma (HCC)?

A. HCC is more rapidly growing than other tumors such as colon and bronchogenic carcinomas.
B. In the United States, the average survival after resection is 3 years and 5-year survival rates after surgery (including transplantation) are between 10 and 50%.
C. The operative mortality is 5 to 10%.

D. Retrospective reviews suggest that in HCC patients with cirrhosis or lesions smaller than 5 cm, transplantation doubles the chance for survival.
E. Most deaths following transplantation for HCC are attributable to liver failure.

DISCUSSION: Retrospective reviews suggest that in HCC patients with cirrhosis or lesions smaller than 5 cm, transplantation doubles the chance for survival versus resection. HCC is a slower-growing tumor than colon cancer or bronchogenic carcinoma. In the United States, the average survival after resection is reported to be approximately 3 years and 5-year survival rates after resection (including liver transplantation) in several large series varied from 11 to 46%. Currently, the operative mortality in the United States is approximately 1%. Most deaths after transplantation for HCC are attributable to tumor recurrence.
Textbook: Page 1028 ANSWER: D

19. Which of the following statements is true in the management of metastatic hepatic malignancies?

A. Without treatment, 60 to 70% of patients with colorectal metastatic liver lesions will die within 1 year.
B. The 5-year survival rate following resection of a solitary colorectal liver metastasis is less than 30%.
C. Contraindications to resection include large symptomatic lesions, total hepatic involvement, advanced jaundice, and vena caval or main portal vein invasion.
D. Survival rates correlate with the interval between resection of the primary lesion and resection of the hepatic metastasis.
E. Patients with multiple metastatic lesions in the same lobe have lower survival rates than those with single lesions.

DISCUSSION: Without treatment, 60 to 70% of patients with colorectal liver metastases die within 1 year and close to 100% die within 3 years. Resection of a solitary metastatic lesion from a colorectal primary tumor can have as much as a 50% 5-year survival rate. In general, contraindications to major hepatic resection for metastatic disease include total hepatic involvement, advanced cirrhosis, jaundice (except from extrinsic hepatic ductal obstruction), or main portal vein invasion, and extrahepatic tumor involvement. Although previously considered unresectable, large lesions may be resected following neoadjuvant chemotherapy with reduction of size. Survival does not correlate with the time interval between resection of the primary tumor and resection of the metastatic tumor, nor with the number of lesions within the same lobe.
Textbook: Page 1030 ANSWER: A

20. Which of the following statements is true regarding benign hepatic neoplasms?

A. Hepatic adenomas are usually multiple and can reach a diameter of 30 cm.
B. Unlike with adenomas, patients with focal nodular hyperplasia (FNH) are usually asymptomatic.
C. Hemorrhage, necrosis, and malignant change are more common in FNH than in adenomas.
D. FNH derives its blood supply peripherally, whereas adenomas derive blood supply centrally.
E. Adenomas blend with the surrounding normal hepatic tissue, whereas FNH appears distinct.

DISCUSSION: Adenomas are usually solitary and may vary in size up to 38 cm. In contrast to adenomas, FNH does not produce symptoms; hemorrhage, rupture, or other problems, such as malignant change, are exceedingly rare. FNH derives its blood supply centrally, whereas adenomas derive theirs peripherally. Unlike adenomas, FNH blends with the surrounding normal hepatic parenchyma.
Textbook: Page 1032 ANSWER: B

21. Which statement is true concerning nonparasitic cysts of the liver?

A. Cysts more commonly occur in the left lobe.
B. They are more common in males.
C. A dominant lesion in a patient with polycystic liver disease can be treated by aspiration.
D. Although traumatic cysts are not true cysts, their management is the same.
E. Unlike cystadenocarcinomas, cystadenomas may be treated by aspiration.

DISCUSSION: Cysts may also form as a consequence of trauma or inflammation; however, these are not true cysts, because they have a fibrous rather than an epithelial lining. There are no special aspects in the treatment of these cysts. Nonparasitic hepatic cysts more commonly occur in the right lobe, and occur four times more commonly in females than in males. The surgical procedure of choice for a symptomatic dominant cyst in polycystic disease is the fenestration operation, in which the symptomatic cyst is made to communicate with the peritoneal cavity. Simple aspiration is a temporizing maneuver. Cystadenomas are difficult to differentiate from cystadenocarcinomas, and therefore should be treated similarly with resection.
Textbook: Page 1033 ANSWER: D

22. Which of the following treatments for bleeding varices best preserves portal blood flow to the liver?

A. Side-to-side portacaval shunt.
B. Transjugular intrahepatic portal systemic shunt (TIPS).
C. Distal splenorenal shunt.
D. Interposition mesocaval shunt with a 16-mm Dacron graft.

DISCUSSION: Choices A, B, and D are all nonselective shunts that completely divert portal blood flow away from the liver. Although each of these shunts was designed to decompress varices as well as preserve some hepatic portal perfusion, experience has shown that the resistance through the shunt is considerably less than through the hepatic sinusoidal bed. Although these nonselective shunts effectively prevent bleeding from varices, they all have a fairly high incidence of post-shunt encephalopathy because of their effect on hepatic portal perfusion. The distal splenorenal shunt separates the splanchnic venous system into two components, a high-pressure superior mesenteric component that continues to perfuse the liver and a decompressed gastrosplenic component that prevents bleeding from varices. Over time, the distal splenorenal shunt also completely diverts portal flow in a fairly high percentage of patients. The attrition in portal flow over time is higher for alcoholic cirrhotic patients than for nonalcoholic cirrhotic patients and for patients with noncirrhotic portal hypertension.

Textbook: Page 1069 ANSWER: C

23. Which of the following pharmacologic agents has been shown to significantly decrease the likelihood of variceal bleeding in patients who have not previously bled (prophylactic treatment)?

A. Vasopressin plus nitroglycerin.
B. Nonselective beta-blocker.
C. Octreotide.
D. Glypressin.

DISCUSSION: Nonselective beta-blockade has been shown to reduce the likelihood of an initial variceal hemorrhage in patients with large varices by about 40%. Several randomized, controlled trials have shown a consistent and significant benefit to this treatment. All of the other choices are drugs that are effective to some degree in controlling acute variceal bleeding, but none of them play a role in long-term treatment of patients with varices.

Textbook: Page 1067 ANSWER: B

24. Which of the following treatments is most effective in both preventing recurrent variceal bleeding and relieving medically intractable ascites?

A. End-to-side portacaval shunt.
B. Distal splenorenal shunt.
C. Esophagogastric devascularization combined with splenectomy.
D. Side-to-side portacaval shunt.

DISCUSSION: All side-to-side shunts—which include the side-to-side portacaval shunt, the transjugular intrahepatic portal systemic shunt (TIPS), and large-bore interposition shunts—decompress the splanchnic venous system and the intrahepatic sinusoidal network, both major sites of ascites formation. Therefore, one of these shunts is preferable for the patient who has bled from varices and who also has difficult-to-manage ascites. One of the objectives of the distal splenorenal shunt is to maintain splanchnic venous hypertension and intrahepatic sinusoidal hypertension. Therefore, the distal splenorenal shunt tends to aggravate rather than relieve ascites. The end-to-side portacaval shunt effectively decompresses the splanchnic venous system, but intrahepatic sinusoidal hypertension may be maintained by hepatic arterial perfusion of the liver and some patients continue to produce ascites. Esophagogastric devascularization combined with splenectomy separates gastric and esophageal varices from the high-pressure splanchnic venous system, but does not decompress either the liver or the splanchnic venous network.

Textbook: Page 1069 ANSWER: D

25. The factor that best correlates with mortality after an operation to prevent variceal bleeding is:

A. Child's class.
B. Emergency surgical intervention.
C. The number of prior variceal bleeding episodes.
D. Age of the patient.

DISCUSSION: The original Child's class is composed of two laboratory tests: serum bilirubin and serum albumin; and three clinical variables: ascites, encephalopathy, and nutrition. Because nutrition is difficult to assess in many patients, this variable has been replaced by the prothrombin time in one modification (Child-Pugh classification). Child's class correlates directly with the probability of mortality after an operation in a patient with advanced liver disease. Mortality rate is less than 5% for Child's Class A, 5 to 15% for Child's Class B, and greater than 15% in Child's Class C. Although the emergency setting, because of persistent variceal bleeding, may worsen the Child's class, it is the Child's class rather than the emergency nature of the procedure that determines postoperative mortality. The number of prior variceal hemorrhages and age of the patient have failed to correlate with mortality after surgical procedures to prevent subsequent variceal bleeding.

Textbook: Page 1062 ANSWER: A

26. A 62-year-old man presents to the emergency room with right upper quadrant abdominal pain, a fever of 39°C, and shaking chills. An ultrasound scan demonstrates gallstones and a dilated common bile duct (1.2 cm) containing a gallstone. The most appropriate antibiotic for empirical treatment in this patient would be:

A. Vancomycin.
B. Metronidazole.
C. Piperacillin/tazobactam.
D. Gentamicin.
E. Ampicillin.

DISCUSSION: This patient has cholangitis secondary to choledocholithiasis. In this setting, *Escherichia coli*, *Klebsiella*, enterococci, and *Bacteroides fragilis* are the most common isolates. Empirical therapy should be selected to cover these organisms. Only piperacillin/tazobactam provides good activity against each of these organisms.

Textbook: Page 1080 ANSWER: C

27. A 50-year-old woman presents to her internist with a 1-week history of jaundice. The internist obtained a liver function panel, which included the following test results: total bilirubin, 6.0 mg/dl; direct bilirubin, 4.7 mg/dl; aspartate aminotransferase (AST), 90 units; alanine aminotransferase (ALT), 75 units; alkaline phosphatase, 445 units. The most appropriate diagnostic study would be a(n):

A. Ultrasound.
B. Liver biopsy.
C. Hepatitis B and C serologies.
D. Magnetic resonance cholangiogram (MRC).
E. Indirect Coombs test.

DISCUSSION: The liver function panel is most compatible with obstructive jaundice from extrahepatic biliary obstruction. Ultrasound offers the most widely available, cost-effective means of documenting the presence of intra- and/or extrahepatic biliary obstruction. In addition, ultrasound can identify gallstones with high sensitivity. MRC is less widely available and in most centers is more costly. However, MRC can also accurately identify the presence of biliary obstruction.

Textbook: Page 1081 ANSWER: A

28. Which of the following statements about cholesterol gallstone pathogenesis is true?

A. Cholesterol gallstones are more common in elderly women (> 65 years of age) than in women in their fourth and fifth decades (30s and 40s).
B. Bile is concentrated in the gallbladder, leading to an increase in the stability of cholesterol-phospholipid vesicles.
C. Cholesterol is highly insoluble in aqueous solutions and is maintained in solution in bile by phospholipids and bilirubin.
D. Cholesterol precipitates more rapidly in bile from patients with gallstones because of several nucleating factors, including deoxycholic acid and bilirubin diglucuronide.

DISCUSSION: The incidence of gallstones increases with age. Concentration of bile in the gallbladder decreases cholesterol-phospholipid vesicle stability. Cholesterol is maintained in solution by phospholipids and bile salts. Nucleating factors in bile include mucin glycoproteins, immunoglobulins, and transferrin.

Textbook: Page 1084 ANSWER: A

29. A 50-year-old man presents to the emergency room with a 24-hour history of right upper quadrant abdominal pain. On physical examination, his abdomen is soft with moderate right subcostal tenderness. He has a fever of 38.5°C. A liver function panel is normal. The most appropriate next study is:

A. Endoscopic retrograde cholangiopancreatography (ERCP).
B. Abdominal ultrasound.
C. Diagnostic laparoscopy.
D. Endoscopic ultrasound.
E. Cholescintigraphy.

DISCUSSION: The most likely diagnosis in this patient with acute right upper quadrant pain and tenderness is acute calculous cholecystitis. An abdominal ultrasound is very sensitive in documenting the presence of gallstones, as well as in confirming the diagnosis of acute cholecystitis. Ultrasound findings consistent with acute cholecystitis include gallbladder wall thickening, pericholecystic fluid, and a sonographic Murphy's sign. Cholescintigraphy is also highly sensitive in diagnosing acute cholecystitis. However, it is more time-consuming, provides less anatomic detail than ultrasound, and is not capable of identifying the presence of gallstones.

Textbook: Page 1086 ANSWER: B

30. One week following a laparoscopic cholecystomy, a 40-year-old woman presents with increasing right upper quadrant pain. A computed tomography scan demonstrates a 10-cm subhepatic fluid collection, and an endoscopic retrograde cholangiopancreatography demonstrates extravasation from the cystic duct. The next appropriate step is:

A. Laparotomy, ligation of the cystic duct, and placement of a subhepatic drain.
B. Laparoscopic drain placement.
C. Percutaneous drainage of fluid collection and placement of an endoprosthesis.
D. Roux-en-Y hepaticojejunostomy.

DISCUSSION: Appropriate management of this patient's biloma and cystic duct bile leak includes drainage of the fluid collection and decompression of the biliary tract until the cystic duct leak is closed. This can be accomplished nonoperatively with percutaneous drainage and placement of an endoprosthesis in the majority of cases.

Textbook: Page 219 ANSWER: C

31. The risk of cholangiocarcinoma is not increased in patients with:

A. Choledochal cyst.
B. Primary sclerosing cholangitis.
C. Hepatolithiasis.
D. Gallstones.
E. *Clonorchis sinensis*.

DISCUSSION: Choledochal cysts, primary sclerosing cholangitis, hepatolithiasis, and *C. sinensis* infection are all associated with an increased risk of cholangiocarcinoma. Gallstones are associated with an increased risk of gallbladder cancer, not cholangiocarcinoma.

Textbook: Page 1105 ANSWER: D

32. A healthy 60-year-old man undergoes an uncomplicated laparoscopic cholecystectomy. The pathologist identifies a gallbladder cancer extending through the lamina propria and muscularis into the serosa. The most appropriate treatment would include:

A. Weekly 5-fluorouracil (5-FU) for 1 year.
B. External-beam radiation therapy to the gallbladder fossa and liver.
C. Resection of liver segments IV and V and lymph node dissection.
D. No further therapy.

DISCUSSION: This pathologic Stage II (T2) gallbladder cancer has a 50% probability of lymph node metastases. Removal of the regional lymph nodes including the cystic duct, pericholedochal, portal, right celiac, and posterior pancreaticoduodenal lymph nodes should be performed. Extension into hepatic parenchyma is common, and "extended cholecystectomy" is performed if a wedge resection of the liver is chosen, or for larger tumors an anatomic liver resection may be required to achieve a histologically negative margin. Response rates to 5-FU are low for gallbladder cancer, and external-beam radiation therapy has not been shown to extend survival in patients with incompletely resected gallbladder cancer.

Textbook: Page 1104 ANSWER: C

33. During a laparotomy for a stab wound to the abdomen two injuries are identified: a gastric laceration and a near-total transection of the tail of the pancreas 2 cm away from the splenic hilum. The most appropriate method of treatment for the pancreatic injury is:

A. Débridement and omental patching.
B. Distal pancreatectomy at the level of the transection.
C. The pyloric exclusion procedure.
D. Extended pancreaticoduodenectomy.
E. Closure of the proximal pancreas and drainage of the distal pancreas to a roux-en-Y limb of jejunum.

DISCUSSION: The most appropriate treatment for a Class III injury to the tail of the pancreas is distal pancreatectomy, which includes the site of the injury. Débridement and omental patching are used for lesser injuries. Both the pyloric exclusion procedure and pancreaticoduodenectomy are used for Class IV severe, combined injuries to the pancreas and duodenum. In the scenario discussed, answer E is incorrect because an attempt to salvage the small amount of pancreatic tissue between the site of the stab wound and the spleen serves no purpose, and exposes the patient to the risk of a pancreatic fistula.

Textbook: Page 335 ANSWER: B

34. Which of the following patients is at the highest personal risk for adenocarcinoma of the pancreas?

A. A woman with three first-degree relatives with the diagnosis of pancreatic cancer.
B. A man with a 60 pack-year history of cigarette smoking.
C. A woman with familial adenomatous polyposis (FAP).
D. A 30-year-old male alcoholic with steatorrhea and midepigastric abdominal pain.
E. A multiparous woman taking birth control pills.

DISCUSSION: Risk factors for pancreatic adenocarcinoma include familial aggregation, tobacco exposure (cigarette smoking,) chronic pancreatitis, and many others. FAP is certainly a known risk factor for colorectal cancer, and it may be a low-level risk factor for pancreatic cancer. Of all the risk factors listed in this question, the presence of three first-degree relatives with pancreatic adenocarcinoma is the highest risk factor, raising the personal risk at least 33-fold over baseline.

Textbook: Page 1133 ANSWER: A

35. A 75-year-old woman is admitted to the hospital with her first episode of gallstone pancreatitis. She is hemodynamically stable, but has severe pain and hypoxemia. Abdominal ultrasound reveals gallbladder stones and a normal common bile duct. Laboratory values at admission are glucose, 250 mg/dl; lactate dehydrogenase (LDH), 500 U/L; aspartate aminotransferase (AST), 300 U/L; amylase, 5000 U/L; total bilirubin, 1.5 mg/dl; and white blood cell count (WBC), 20,000 mm^3. Which of the following is the best management strategy?

A. Admit to the intensive care unit (ICU) setting, fluid-resuscitate, and begin antibiotics.
B. Admit to the ICU setting, fluid-resuscitate, and plan urgent laparoscopic cholecystectomy plus laparoscopic common bile duct exploration.
C. Admit to the ICU setting, fluid-resuscitate, begin histamine-2 (H_2)-antagonist and atropine therapy.
D. Admit to nonmonitored bed, and perform urgent percutaneous transhepatic cholangiography (PTC) and stone extraction.
E. Admit to nonmonitored bed, begin peritoneal dialysis, and administer ursodiol (Actigall).

DISCUSSION: The patient presented has gallstone pancreatitis and five Ranson prognostic signs (age, WBC, glucose, LDH, and AST) at admission. She would therefore be classified as having severe pancreatitis. She should be admitted to an ICU setting for proper monitoring, receive intravenous fluids and analgesics, and be started on antibiotics for prophylaxis against septic complications. Laparoscopic cholecystectomy is normally delayed until clinical improvement occurs. Neither H_2-antagonist nor atropine therapy has proved to be of benefit. Although controversial in regard to timing and indications, the safest route for study of the biliary tree and stone extraction is endoscopic (via endoscopic retrograde cholangiopancreatography and sphincterotomy, not percutaneous (via PTC).

Textbook: Page 1121 ANSWER: A

36. A 35-year-old man with a long history of alcohol abuse has progressive constant midepigastric pain and normal liver function tests. His evaluation includes abdominal computed tomography, showing a calcified pancreas, no evidence of biliary dilatation, and a markedly dilated main pancreatic duct. Initial recommendations are for cessation of alcohol use and pancreatic enzyme supplementation. Three months later he continues to have pain requiring narcotic analgesics. The most appropriate surgical intervention would be:

A. Celiac denervation, to include vagotomy.
B. Distal pancreatectomy with splenic preservation.
C. Distal pancreatectomy with splenectomy.
D. Transduodenal biliary sphincteroplasty with pancreatic duct septoplasty.
E. Longitudinal pancreaticojejunostomy.

DISCUSSION: Longitudinal pancreaticoduodenectomy (Peustow procedure) is a ductal decompressive procedure that appears to be ideal for patients with chronic pancreatitis and a markedly dilated pancreatic duct. Such a procedure avoids pancreatic resection and maximally preserves both endocrine and exocrine function. In general, resectional procedures are avoided if ductal drainage procedures are applicable. Celiac denervation plus vagotomy is unlikely to give long-lasting pain relief, and may be associated with gastric motility problems. Ampullary procedures (such as sphincteroplasty and septoplasty) typically do not improve patients with chronic pancreatitis.

Textbook: Page 1127 ANSWER: E

37. A fit 72-year-old man develops obstructive jaundice, with a total bilirubin of 12 mg/dl. Abdominal computed tomography reveals dilated intrahepatic and extrahepatic bile ducts, a distended gallbladder, and a 2-cm hypodense mass in the head of the pancreas. Prior to exploration, work-up *must* include which of the following?

A. Staging laparoscopy.
B. Serum amylase, carcinoembryonic antigen (CEA) and CA 19–9.
C. Coagulation parameters.
D. Endoscopic retrograde cholangiopancreatography (ERCP) with stent placement.
E. Magnetic resonance cholangiopancreatography (MRCP).

DISCUSSION: In this setting, prior to exploration it is mandatory that coagulation parameters (prothrombin time [PT], partial thromboplastin time) be checked and normalized. Obstructive jaundice may be associated with prolongation of the PT due to malabsorption of vitamin K. Although staging laparoscopy is used by some surgeons to stage patients with presumed cancer of the head of the pancreas, its use is not mandatory or universal. Blood tests such as serum amylase, CEA, and CA 19–9 may or may not be evaluated, and often have little impact on therapy. ERCP with stent placement is not mandatory in this patient, nor is MRCP.

Textbook: Page 1134 ANSWER: C

38. The visceral relationships of the spleen are with all of the following except:

A. The greater curvature of the stomach.
B. The tail of the pancreas.
C. The left kidney.
D. The third portion of the duodenum.
E. The splenic flexure of the colon.

DISCUSSION: The visceral relationships of the spleen are with the proximal greater curvature of the stomach, the tail of the pancreas, the left kidney, and the splenic flexure of the colon. The third portion of the duodenum is separated from the spleen by the transverse colon and mesocolon and the root of the small bowel mesentery.

Textbook: Page 1145 ANSWER: D

39. Normal functions of the adult spleen include all of the following except:

A. Hematopoiesis.
B. Erythrocyte processing and repair.
C. Production of opsonins.
D. Destruction of aged and damaged erythrocytes.
E. Clearance of circulating bacteria.

DISCUSSION: The normal functions of the adult spleen include all of those listed except hematopoiesis. Although hematopoiesis is an important function of the spleen during early fetal development, with both red and white blood cell production, there is no significant hematopoietic function remaining by the fifth month of gestation. Only under certain pathologic conditions such as myelodysplasia does the spleen reacquire its hematopoietic function in the adult.

Textbook: Page 1144 ANSWER: A

40. Appropriate initial treatment for the patient with idiopathic thrombocytopenic purpura (ITP) includes which of the following?

A. Observation alone for asymptomatic patients with platelet counts above 50,000 mm^3.
B. Hospitalization and platelet transfusion for an asymptomatic patient with a platelet count of 30,000 mm^3.
C. Low-dose aspirin therapy to prevent thrombotic complications.
D. Azathioprine.
E. None of the above.

DISCUSSION: Observation alone for asymptomatic patients with platelet counts above 50,000 mm^3 is the appropriate initial treatment. Neither hospitalization nor platelet transfusion is necessary for the asymptomatic patient with a platelet count of 30,000 mm^3. Patients with platelet counts greater than 20,000 mm^3 do not require hospitalization if they are asymptomatic or have only minor purpura. Hospitalization is often required for patients with platelet counts of less than 20,000 mm^3 who have significant mucous membrane bleeding or severe life-threatening hemorrhage. Platelet transfusion is seldom indicated in pa-

tients with ITP in the absence of severe hemorrhage. Aspirin is containdicated in patients with thrombocytopenia because it inhibits platelet function. Azathioprine is sometimes used as treatment for ITP patients who fail to achieve adequate response after splenectomy.
Textbook: Page 1147 ANSWER: A

41. All of the following are true statements except:
A. Splenectomy is indicated for patients with non-Hodgkin's lymphoma with symptomatic splenomegaly.
B. Improved imaging techniques have decreased the numbers of patients with Hodgkin's disease requiring staging laparotomy.
C. Splenectomy is the optimal initial treatment for patients with hairy cell leukemia and moderate splenomegaly.
D. Approximately 40% of patients with hairy cell leukemia have normalization of their blood counts after splenectomy.
E. Splenectomy has not resulted in improved survival in patients receiving allogeneic bone marrow transplantation for chronic myeloid leukemia (CML).

DISCUSSION: Although splenectomy and alpha$_2$-interferon have been standard treatment of hairy cell leukemia until recently, this approach is being replaced with systemic administration of purine analogues such as 2-chlorodeoxyadenosine or deoxycoformycin as initial treatment. Splenectomy is still indicated for some patients with massive enlargement of the spleen or with evidence of hypersplenism that is refractory to medical therapy. All of the other statements are true.
Textbook: Pages 1149–1151 ANSWER: C

NOTES

NOTES

CHAPTER 13

CHEST

1. The most common cause of mediastinitis is:

A. Esophageal rupture.
B. Mediastinoscopy.
C. Tracheobronchial perforation.
D. Postoperative following median sternotomy for cardiac surgery.
E. Mediastinal extension from an infectious process originating in the pulmonary parenchyma.

DISCUSSION: Mediastinitis occurs most often after median sternotomy for open heart cardiac operations. Superficial wound infections occur in approximately 4% of patients after cardiac operations; in 1 to 2% of patients the infection involves the mediastinum. The risk factors for the development of mediastinitis include prolonged operation, obesity, lengthy cardiopulmonary bypass, re-exploration for postoperative bleeding, dehiscence, external cardiac massage, postoperative cardiogenic shock, and the use of bilateral internal mammary arteries for coronary artery bypass grafting, especially in elderly patients or in patients with diabetes mellitus.

Textbook: Page 1185 ANSWER: D

2. A 25-year-old man presents to his internist with complaints of dyspnea, cough, and chest discomfort. His physical examination is unremarkable, but chest radiograph shows a large anterior mediastinal mass. The most appropriate next step in his treatment would be:

A. Serologic measurements of alpha-fetoprotein and beta-human chorionic gonadotropin (β-HCG).
B. Admit and place the patient on intravenous antibiotics.
C. Begin chemotherapy.
D. Order an arteriogram to assess for vascular invasion.
E. Send the patient home with follow-up in 1 week.

DISCUSSION: Malignant germ cell tumors also occur predominantly in the anterosuperior mediastinum. Unlike benign teratomas, there is a marked male predominance. The peak incidence is in the third and fourth decades of life. The majority of patients are symptomatic with chest pain, cough, dyspnea, and hemoptysis; the superior vena caval syndrome occurs commonly. The chest film usually demonstrates a large anterior mediastinal mass that is often multilobular. Serologic measurements of alpha-fetoprotein and β-HCG are useful for the following tasks: differentiating seminomas from nonseminomas, quantitatively assessing response to therapy in hormonally active tumors (plasma half-life of alpha-fetoprotein and β-HCG is 5 days and 12 to 24 hours, respectively), and diagnosing relapse or failure of therapy before changes that can be observed in gross disease. Seminomas rarely produce β-HCG (<7%) and never produce alpha-fetoprotein; in contrast, over 90% of nonseminomas secrete one or both of these hormones. This differentiation is important because of the marked radiosensitivity of seminomas and the relative radiosensitivity of nonseminomas. Serologic evaluation is indicated in certain patients. Male patients with an anterosuperior mediastinal mass in the second through fifth decades should have alpha-fetoprotein and β-HCG serologies obtained. A positive serology is indicative of a nonseminomatous germ cell tumor.

Textbook: Page 1188 ANSWER: A

3. The three most common mediastinal tumors found in adults, excluding cysts, are:

A. Thymomas, germ cell tumors, neurogenic tumors.
B. Thymomas, mesenchymal tumors, germ cell tumors.
C. Neurogenic tumors, thymomas, lymphomas.
D. Lymphomas, parathyroid adenomas, thyroid adenomas.
E. Neurogenic tumors, thymomas, mesenchymal tumors.

DISCUSSION: Although differences in the relative incidence of neoplasms exist in some series, the most common mediastinal masses are neurogenic tumors (20%), thymomas (19%), and lymphomas (13%).

Textbook: Pages 1188–1189 ANSWER: C

4. A 28-year-old woman presents with complaints of malaise, low-grade fevers, and increasing dyspnea. Physical examination is unremarkable, and chest radiographs show the presence of a mediastinal mass near the hilum of the left lung. Computed tomography scan confirms the presence of a 3 × 4 cm left hilar mass, but additionally the presence of diffuse paratracheal adenopathy is noted. The best approach to obtaining tissue for diagnosis would be:

A. Mediastinoscopy.
B. Median sternotomy.
C. Posterolateral thoracotomy.
D. Clam-shell incision.
E. No tissue necessary, as the likelihood of this being a lymphoma is high enough that treatment can be instituted without pathologic confirmation.

DISCUSSION: Mediastinoscopy is a useful technique to evaluate and biopsy lesions of the middle mediastinum. Often this technique is used to evaluate associated lymphadenopathy in this region. Lesions in the anterosuperior mediastinum that are unresectable are best biopsied using a limited anterior second or third interspace parasternal mediastinotomy or using thoracoscopy. Similarly, unresectable lesions in the superior mediastinum, hilar, or paratracheal regions can be sampled through a small lateral thoracotomy in the third or fourth interspace after retracting the apex of the lung inferiorly. Unresectable posterior mediastinal masses may be approached thoracoscopically or through a limited posterolateral thoracotomy.

Textbook: Page 1189 ANSWER: A

5. Primary germ cell tumors of the mediastinum:

A. Have a better prognosis than their gonadal counterparts.
B. Show a marked male predominance for the nonseminomatous tumors.
C. Are always malignant.
D. Most commonly present as asymptomatic masses.
E. Are universally fatal.

DISCUSSION: Germ cell tumors of the mediastinum are benign and malignant neoplasms thought to originate from primordial germ cells that fail to complete the migration from the urogenital ridge and come to rest in the mediastinum. Germ cell tumors occur predominantly in the anterosuperior mediastinum. Unlike benign teratomas, malignant germ cell tumors show a marked male predominance. The peak incidence is in the third and fourth decades of life. The majority of patients are symptomatic with chest pain, cough, dyspnea, and hemoptysis; the superior vena caval syndrome occurs commonly.

Textbook: Page 1195 ANSWER: B

6. A 48-year-old woman with myasthenia gravis is found on computed tomography scanning to have a thymoma. Which of the following is a true statement?

A. Patients with myasthenia gravis have a higher postoperative mortality than their nonmyasthenic counterparts.
B. In this patient population thymomas are always malignant.
C. Thymectomy results in a complete remission of myasthenic symptoms in almost 100% of patients.
D. Maximization of perioperative management is vital in decreasing morbidity from surgery.
E. Medical treatment without thymectomy is recommended for the majority of patients.

DISCUSSION: Although myasthenic patients with thymoma had a worse prognosis in past series, improvements in therapy for myasthenia gravis have allowed prognosis to be dependent on the stage of the disease rather than on the presence of myasthenia gravis. In patients with myasthenia gravis, perioperative patient management is extremely important to prevent complications. Anticholinesterase inhibitors are discontinued to decrease the amount of pulmonary secretions and prevent inadvertent cholinergic weakness. Plasmapheresis is used routinely within 72 hours of thymectomy. In the majority of patients, plasmapheresis is very effective in controlling generalized weakness. Also, careful attention to the maintenance of pulmonary function with chest physiotherapy, endotracheal suctioning, and bronchodilators is the mainstay of postoperative management. The decision to extubate is based on evidence of adequate respiratory mechanics (e.g., vital capacity > 15 ml/kg and expiratory pressures > 40 cm H_2O) rather than evidence of adequate ventilation, as determined by analysis of arterial blood gases.

Textbook: Page 1195 ANSWER: D

7. The superior vena caval syndrome is:

A. Most commonly seen with benign tumors in adults.
B. Uniformly fatal.
C. Caused by tumors that are frequently surgically resectable.
D. Rare in thin patients.
E. An occasional presentation of many mediastinal tumors as well as bronchogenic carcinoma.

DISCUSSION: A number of benign and malignant processes may cause obstruction of the superior vena cava, leading to superior vena caval syndrome. The pathophysiology of the syndrome involves the increased pressure in the venous system draining into the superior vena cava, producing the characteristic features of the syndrome, which include edema of the head, neck, and upper extremities; distended neck veins with dilated collateral veins over the upper extremities and torso; cyanosis; headache; and confusion. Superior vena caval obstruction may arise from compression, invasion, or thrombosis. The cause may be the primary tumor or mass or is often due to paratracheal lymph node metastases. Whereas in adults the most frequent cause is a malignant neoplasm, in children a bronchogenic carcinoma is the usual etiology. The syndrome is most common after cardiac surgical procedures, particularly atrial level repairs for transposition of the great vessels. Rarely are the malignant processes responsible for the superior vena caval syndrome surgically resectable.

Textbook: Page 1186 ANSWER: E

8. An 11-month-old boy develops fevers, cough, strange darting eye movements, and becomes notably more irritable. During evaluation a chest radiograph is obtained which shows a posterior mediastinal mass. The most likely diagnosis is:

A. Thymoma.
B. Enteric cyst.
C. Neuroblastoma.
D. Lymphoma.
E. Primary lung carcinoma.

DISCUSSION: Neuroblastomas originate from the sympathetic nervous system. The most common location for a neuroblastoma is in the retroperitoneum; however, 10 to 20% occur primarily in the mediastinum. These are highly invasive neoplasms that have frequently metastasized before diagnosis. Common sites of metastases are the regional lymph nodes, bone, brain, liver, and lung. A majority of these tumors occur in children, and 75% occur in children <4 years of age. The tumor is composed of small, round, immature cells organized in a rosette pattern. On ultrastructural examination, the presence of neurosecretory granules is characteristic. Patients are usually symptomatic. A variety of paraneoplastic syndromes have been reported, including profuse watery diarrhea and abdominal pain related to vasoactive intestinal polypeptide production, the opsoclonus-polymyoclonus syndrome (an unexplained symptom complex characterized by cerebellar and truncal ataxia with rapid, darting eye movements [dancing eyes] that is possibly related to an autoimmune mechanism), and pheochromocytoma syndrome due to catecholamine secretion.

Textbook: Page 1190 ANSWER: C

9. A 70-year-old man was noted to have a 3.5-cm mass centrally located in the right upper lobe on a chest roentgenogram. Computed tomography (CT) of the chest (including the liver and adrenals) was performed. The right upper lobe mass was confirmed and a 1.5-cm right paratracheal lymph node was identified. No other abnormalities were noted. The clinical stage of this patient is:

A. IB.
B. IIA.
C. IIB.
D. IIIA.
E. IIIB.

DISCUSSION: The preoperative evaluation of the patient with a suspected lung cancer requires the surgeon to determine the extent of the disease and if surgery can be performed safely. The preoperative clinical stage of the patient suggests the appropriate treatment. In this patient, the clinical stage is based on the size of the primary tumor and the identification of enlarged ($\geq$ 1.0 cm) right paratracheal lymph nodes. The T descriptor would be T2 and the N descriptor would be N2. No metastases (M0) were identified. (In the absence of neurologic symptoms or bone pain, CT [or magnetic resonance imaging] brain or bone scan [respectively] would not be required.) The patient has a T2N2M0 clinical stage IIIA lung cancer.

Textbook: Page 1216 ANSWER: D

10. The patient should next undergo:

A. Fine-needle aspiration of the right upper lobe mass.
B. Bronchoscopy.
C. Mediastinoscopy.
D. Bronchoscopy and mediastinoscopy.
E. Lobectomy and mediastinal lymph node sampling / dissection.

DISCUSSION: Evaluation would include bronchoscopy and mediastinoscopy. If the patient were not a surgical candidate, fine-needle aspiration would be appropriate to determine the histology of the cancer prior to initiating other alternative treatment modalities (such as chemotherapy and radiation therapy). If metastases to N2 lymph nodes were identified by mediastinoscopy, the patient could be considered for entry into prospective protocols evaluating chemotherapy and radiation and surgery for treatment. Alternatively, chemotherapy and radiation could be considered for definitive therapy.

Textbook: Page 1217 ANSWER: D

11. After resection, pathologic examination of the specimen revealed a 3.7-cm adenocarcinoma of the right upper lobe. Two of five lymph nodes in the hilum were positive for adenocarcinoma. One of seven 4R were positive for adenocarcinoma. All other lymph nodes (levels 1, 7, 8, 9) were negative. No other metastases were noted. The pathologic stage of this patient is:

A. IB.
B. IIA.
C. IIB.
D. IIIA.
E. IIIB.

DISCUSSION: The pathologic descriptors demonstrate a T2 (3.7-cm tumor size), N2 (positive-level, four lymph nodes) M0 adenocarcinoma: pathologic stage IIIA (T2N2M0). If the patient did not have preoperative therapy, radiation therapy could be considered to enhance local tumor control.

Textbook: Page 1216 ANSWER: D

12. A patient was found to have pulmonary metastasis after treatment for a primary tumor. Indications for resection of pulmonary metastasis include all of the following except:

A. Prior wide local excision of a malignant fibrous histiocytoma of the thigh.
B. Eight pulmonary nodules (ranging in size from 0.3 to 1.7 cm) in a patient with a previous synovial cell sarcoma.
C. Predicted postoperative FEV_1 of 0.9 L.
D. Solitary hepatic metastasis (left lateral segment) in a patient with a colorectal cancer.
E. Hilar tumor encasing the right main

pulmonary artery at the level of the truncus anterior and a large 8-cm left lower lobe metastasis.

DISCUSSION: In a patient with sarcoma, the primary tumor is usually well controlled with a wide local excision. The number of pulmonary nodules, eight, is not by itself a contraindication for surgery. If the patient is completely resectable based on the evaluation by the surgeon, surgery is appropriately indicated. The surgeon must consider that sarcomas frequently (approximately 50%) have occult metastases that are not detectable even with high-resolution computed tomography scans. In some centers, chemotherapy is used to evaluate biologic response in patients with multiple pulmonary metastases. If a biologic response is identified (decrease in tumor size, decreasing tumor number, etc.), then chemotherapy is continued until the disease is stabilized. Surgery is then performed for "salvage" treatment of residual disease.

In patients with pulmonary metastasis from colorectal carcinoma, a solitary hepatic metastasis that is easily resectable is not a contraindication to surgery. Resection of the lung metastasis and the liver metastasis may be performed at the same time or, alternatively, they may be performed as staged operations. In this situation, the hepatic operation is typically done first to optimize the patient's postoperative recovery and lung function during that recovery. The pulmonary metastasis is then resected afterward.

A postoperative predicted FEV_1 of 0.9 L is sufficient for independent activity without oxygen. A patient would require a pneumonectomy on one side, and a lobectomy on the other would not provide sufficient residual pulmonary reserve to sustain independent existence.

Selection of patients for resection of pulmonary metastasis is based on broad criteria. These criteria are sufficiently broad so as not to exclude patients who could conceivably benefit from resection of their metastasis. Criteria for resection of pulmonary metastasis typically include (a) pulmonary nodules consistent with metastases; (b) control of the primary tumor; (c) all nodules are potentially resectable with a single or staged surgical procedure; (d) adequate postoperative pulmonary reserve; and (e) absence of uncontrolled extrathoracic metastasis.

Other relative indications for resection of pulmonary metastasis include (a) obtain a diagnosis; (b) obtain samples of residual disease after chemotherapy to evaluate treatment effects; (c) obtain tissues for markers, chemosensitivity assays, and immunologic or immunohistochemical studies; and (d) decrease tumor burden.

Textbook: Page 1225 ANSWER: E

13. The most consistent prognostic indicator associated with improved postresection survival in a patient with pulmonary metastases is:

A. Sarcoma histology.
B. Disease-free interval (length of time from date of primary resection to date of identification of pulmonary metastases) of greater than 12 months.
C. Tumor doubling time greater than 20 days.
D. Solitary metastasis.
E. Complete resection.

DISCUSSION: Various clinical factors or prognostic indicators have been examined to evaluate their relationship to survival in patients with pulmonary metastasis. Patients with more virulent tumors tend to have shorter survival times. Various clinical observations may suggest a more aggressive tumor; these include shorter disease-free interval, more rapid tumor doubling time, and multiple unresectable metastases. Patients with pulmonary metastasis may have disease localized to the lungs and they have been shown to benefit from resection of these metastases. In these individuals, complete resection is typically associated with improved survival regardless of histology. In patients who undergo a complete resection, other prognostic indicators may suggest better survival. These more favorable indicators include patients with solitary metastasis, longer tumor doubling times, and longer disease-free intervals. These criteria, however, are relative, and completeness of resection, not number of metastases or disease-free interval or tumor doubling time, should be the critical factor in recommending resection for pulmonary metastases.

Textbook: Page 1226 ANSWER: E

14. All of the following pulmonary function studies suggest a low risk for perioperative morbidity or mortality after pulmonary resection except:

A. Predicted postoperative FEV_1 of 0.810 L.
B. Predicted postoperative FEV_1 of 40%.
C. Cigarette smoking cessation 9 weeks prior to surgery.
D. D_LCO is 49% of that predicted.
E. MVO_2 ($\dot{V}O_2$ max) of 9 ml/kg/min.

DISCUSSION: Predictors of increased pulmonary morbidity are varied and measure various aspects of pulmonary, cardiac, and cardiopulmonary function. Spirometry and arterial blood gases are the simplest and most readily available studies. Patients with a postoperative predicted FEV_1 of less than 0.8 L or less than 40% are at increased risk for pulmonary complications. Patients who are currently smoking should cease smoking prior to surgery. Patients should be smoke-free for a minimum of 2 to 8 weeks prior to pulmonary resection. D_LCO measures the diffusion of carbon monoxide across the alveolar membrane to the alveolar capillary bed. Patients with a D_LCO of less than 40% are at increased risk for pulmonary resection. Patients with an MVO_2 ($\dot{V}O_2$max) of less than 15 ml/kg/min are at prohibitive risk for pulmonary resection.

Textbook: Pages 1206–1208 ANSWER: E

15. A 57-year-old woman has acute lymphocytic leukemia and granulocytopenia following aggressive chemotherapy. A fever and a mild cough prompted a chest x-ray that demonstrated diffuse consolidation in the right upper lobe. Tissue biopsy confirmed the diagnosis of aspergillosis and treatment with antifungal drugs was begun. Three weeks later, hemoptysis occurred only once (500 ml in 24 hours) and follow-up chest x-ray demonstrated a small (1-cm) fungus ball in a 3-cm right upper lobe cavity. Bronchoscopy was unremarkable except for erythema at the orifice of the right upper lobe. The next most appropriate therapy would be:

A. High-dose systemic (intravenous) amphotericin B therapy.
B. Insertion of a percutaneous catheter and irrigation with antifungal agents.
C. Bronchial artery embolization and continuation of antifungal agents.
D. Cavernostomy with removal of the fungus ball.
E. Lobectomy.

DISCUSSION: Pulmonary aspergillosis may occur in three general categories: allergic aspergillosis, colonizing aspergillosis, and invasive aspergillosis. Invasive aspergillosis typically occurs in patients with prolonged and profound granulocytopenia or other attenuation of the immune system. *Aspergillus* is commonly found in decaying vegetation, soil, organic debris, or on stored hay or grain. The organism is inhaled and infects the lungs. Invasive aspergillosis occurs in patients with immunosuppression. After germination, endobronchial proliferation occurs. The bronchial walls may ulcerate; the hyphae may invade pulmonary arterioles. Hemoptysis may occur. Clinical symptoms of fever and bronchitis may be present. A chest x-ray may demonstrate a patchy density or consolidation in the infected lung. Further disruption of the lung parenchyma with necrosis may yield a cavity. Debris may be sequestered and form a fungus ball. The fungus ball can be demonstrated on chest x-ray or computed tomography. Amphotericin B remains the major intravenous agent available. Oral medications such as itraconazole may be considered, although variable absorption and variation of serum levels have been noted. In patients with hemoptysis or local disease, surgical resection may be indicated. Surgical resection controls the disease locally after failure of medical therapy. Systemic therapy should be initiated prior to surgical manipulation. Cavernostomy with removal of the fungus ball would not remove all the infected tissue. Bronchial artery embolization when a patient's hemoptysis has ceased would carry more risk than benefit. Irrigation of the cavity with antifungal agents would not clear the disease, although it may be of some value in patients at high risk for pulmonary resection.

Textbook: Page 1237 ANSWER: A

16. The most frequently used operative technique for repair of pectus excavatum:

A. Requires complete extirpation of the sternum with mirror-image rotation and replacement.
B. Requires entrance into the pleurae for secure surgical repair.
C. Involves both an osteotomy and permanent sternal strut.
D. Gives a good cosmetic result but is followed by recurrence in greater than 50% of patients.

DISCUSSION: The technique that employs an osteotomy and sternal support strut has found the most favor of the surgical repairs. A bioabsorbable strut can be used. Long-term follow up has confirmed excellent patient satisfaction and a low objective rate of recurrence.

Textbook: Page 1168 ANSWER: C

17. The most common tumor of the chest wall is:

A. Fibrous dysplasia.
B. Chondrosarcoma.
C. Metastatic neoplasm.
D. Eosinophilic granuloma.

DISCUSSION: Although chondrosarcoma is the most common malignant chest wall tumor and fibrous dyplasia is the most common benign chest wall lesion, metastatic tumors of the chest wall are at least threefold more common than primary chest wall tumors.

Textbook: Page 1170 ANSWER: C

18. All of the following are true regarding thoracic outlet syndrome (TOS) except:

A. Symptomatology varies widely.
B. Management usually involves surgery.
C. TOS cannot be positively diagnosed on the basis of a single study.
D. It may be precipitated by cold weather or exercise.

DISCUSSION: Symptomatology in TOS is variable based on the structures affected. Cold weather or exercise may induce symptoms in some patients. The initial management of TOS is nonsurgical and involves physical therapy. Many different tests may suggest TOS, but no single result, in isolation, can definitively diagnose TOS.

Textbook: Page 1174 ANSWER: B

19. Pleural effusions:

A. Result from deranged fluid mechanics in the pleural space.
B. Are characterized as exudative if the pleural fluid lactate dehydrogenase (LDH) is >150.
C. May be treated with talc pleurodesis for both malignant and benign etiologies.
D. All begin as transudate.

DISCUSSION: Both benign and malignant pleuralf effusions may be effectively treated wtih talc pleurodesis, although this is generally used in malignant and recurrent or recalcitrant benign effusions. Not all effusions are the results of deranged fluid mechanics or begin as transudates. The serum LDH and control range are important when characterizing pleural effusions.

Textbook: Page 1175 ANSWER: C

20. Surgery for the treatment of pneumothoraces:

A. Is never indicated for a primary spontaneous pneumothorax.
B. Has remained unchanged over the past 25 years.
C. Always involves resection of apical blebs.
D. Is highly effective at preventing recurrence.

DISCUSSION: Surgical treatment of pneumothoraces in numerous studies is found to be effective in >90% of patients. Video-assisted thoracoscopic surgery (VATS) for this disease has become the standard. Several indications for surgical treatment of a primary pneumothorax exist. Surgery often involves resection of apical blebs, but blebs may be found elsewhere in the lung necessitating a thorough search at the time of surgery. Occasionally blebs cannot be identified at surgery and some form of pleurodesis should be carried out.

Textbook: Page 1181 ANSWER: D

21. The following statements regarding mesothelioma are true except:

A. The localized variant is rare.
B. The diffuse variant generally originates in the parietal pleura and spreads to involve the visceral pleura.
C. Conventional chemotherapeutic agents have no activity against mesothelioma.
D. The epithelial subtype shows the most favorable outcome of radical resection.

DISCUSSION: Chemotherapeutic agents have been shown to have moderate activity against mesothelioma, similar to that of non–small cell lung cancer. This activity is less when compared with responses of other types of cancers to chemotherapy.

Textbook: Page 1182 ANSWER: C

NOTES

NOTES

CHAPTER 14

CARDIAC

1. Which of the following statements regarding a patent ductus arteriosus (PDA) is true?

A. Surgical ligation is the treatment of choice in a ventilated, premature infant.
B. Coil occlusion can be safely performed in all adult patients with a PDA.
C. A PDA can be kept open with oral indomethacin.
D. A PDA can be right-sided, or even bilateral.
E. Bacterial endocarditis occurs frequently in adults with a PDA.

DISCUSSION: In a ventilated, premature infant, the treatment of choice is a trial of pharmacological closure of the PDA with indomethacin. Surgical closure in this situation is limited to failure of medical therapy. Catheter coil occlusion, although less invasive, is not suitable for all adult or older patients. Some contraindications include a calcified PDA, an aneurysmal PDA, or a very short or wide PDA relative to the size of the coil. Indomethacin inhibits prostaglandin synthesis and thus promotes ductal closure. Morphologically, a PDA can be right-sided or even bilateral. This reflects the bilateral aortic arch developmental pattern in the embryo. Bacterial endocarditis is fortunately a rare occurrence in patients with a PDA.

Textbook: Page 1244 ANSWER: D

2. In an atrial septal defect (ASD):

A. Eisenmenger's syndrome does not occur due to the low pressure of the shunt at an atrial level.
B. A sinus venosus defect is best corrected in the first 3 months of life.
C. Surgical closure is always indicated.
D. The amount of shunting to the pulmonary bed depends on the difference between the left and right ventricular diastolic pressures.
E. Surgical closure puts the bundle of His at risk.

DISCUSSION: Eisenmenger's syndrome is a result of a raised, fixed pulmonary vascular resistance causing a reversal of flow of the shunt and subsequent cyanosis. The low pressure of the atrial-level shunt in an ASD is unimportant. It is the volume load that leads to an increased pulmonary blood flow, and causes the pulmonary hypertension. An isolated sinus venous defect is not necessarily best corrected in the first 3 months of life. Waiting until the child is older, or in cardiac failure, allows a more accurate surgical repair. Surgical closure of an ASD is not always indicated, as many of these defects may be amenable to transcatheter device closure. In patients more than 60 years of age, there is no documented benefit for routine closure of a hemodynamically insignificant ASD. Physiologically, the amount of blood flow to the pulmonary bed ultimately depends on the difference between the right and left ventricular diastolic pressures. These reflect the mean pressure in the right and left atria. Surgical ASD closure should not routinely put the bundle of His at risk, as this would be away from the area of suture line placement.

Textbook: Page 1245 ANSWER: D

3. Which of the following statements is true concerning the hypoplastic left heart syndrome?

A. It is one of the least frequent congenital cardiac abnormalities encountered.
B. Preoperative stabilization includes prostaglandin E_1 and hyperventilation with 100% oxygen to maintain oxygen saturations above 90%.
C. Associated noncardiac abnormalities are extremely rare.
D. Transplant is a reasonable first-stage option in the management of these patients.
E. The first stage of surgical management is the performance of a bidirectional Glenn shunt.

DISCUSSION: The hypoplastic left heart syndrome and its variants are one of the most frequently encountered groups of congenital abnormalities. By definition, these patients have a physiologic circulation that is in parallel, and preoperative stabilization with 100% oxygen would be fatal in this setting. The key in these patients preoperatively and postoperatively is to balance the circulation, maintaining oxygen saturations around 75 to 80%, thus avoiding excessive pulmonary blood flow and decreased systemic blood flow. Associated noncardiac abnormalities are unfortunately very common. Cardiac transplantation has been documented as a reasonable first-stage option by many centers involved in the management of these infants. The first stage of surgical management is the Norwood procedure or a modification, with a bidirectional Glenn shunt being the intermediary, or second, stage to a Fontan procedure.

Textbook: Page 1260 ANSWER: D

4. Which of the following statements is true about ventricular septal defects (VSDs)?

A. They never close spontaneously, unless they are malalignment defects.
B. They have a lower incidence of subacute bacterial endocarditis (SBE) than atrial septal defects (ASDs).
C. Isolated subarterial defects are best closed through the pulmonary artery.
D. Surgical closure can usually be achieved by direct suture.
E. Aortic valve prolapse is associated with a muscular, inlet type of VSD.

DISCUSSION: Spontaneous closure of VSDs is well documented. Closure or size reduction occurs especially if the defect is not malalignment in nature. The incidence of SBE is higher than that from ASDs, and this is thought to be due to the higher turbulence associated with the increased flow across the VSD. Isolated subarterial defects are easily accessed through the pulmonary artery. Surgical closure usually requires placement of a patch to fill the defect. Direct suture is only rarely employed. Aortic valve prolapse is usually associated with a subarterial defect and is related to a lack of support of the right and noncoronary cusps in the immediate subaortic area. A muscular, inlet type of VSD is remote from the aortic valve, and prolapse is not usually associated with this defect.
Textbook: Page 1246 ANSWER: C

5. Which of the following statements regarding double outlet right ventricle (DORV) is true?

A. The ventricular septal defect (VSD) is always located in a subarterial position.
B. A Fontan approach may be recommended for patients with complex forms of DORV.
C. A conduit between the right ventricle and pulmonary artery is always required for complete repair of DORV with subpulmonary VSD.
D. Neonatal repair is possible in all forms of DORV.
E. In DORV with a subpulmonary VSD, subaortic stenosis and arch obstruction are infrequent.

DISCUSSION: The position of the VSD in DORV is crucial in determining the optimal management strategy. The VSD may be subaortic, subpulmonary, doubly committed, or remote. A single ventricle or Fontan approach for complex types of DORV may be the only way to achieve palliation. Conduit placement between the right ventricle and pulmonary artery is not indicated in DORV with a subpulmonary VSD. The pulmonary artery is not compromised, and the outflow tract is usually unaffected. The issue with the subpulmonary VSD is nearly always the malalignment related to compromise of the aortic outflow. Complete neonatal repair is nearly always impossible in DORV. In patients with a subpulmonary VSD, subaortic stenosis and arch obstruction are frequently encountered.
Textbook: Page 1254 ANSWER: C

6. In simple transposition of the great arteries (TGA), which statement is correct?

A. The procedure of choice is the neonatal atrial switch operation.
B. Ventriculoarterial discordance and atrioventricular discordance are present.
C. Cardiac catheterization is required preoperatively in most cases of simple TGA.
D. The arterial switch operation has a high rate of long-term complications, including baffle obstruction.
E. Simple TGA presents in the neonatal period with cyanosis soon after birth, which becomes worse with ductal closure.

DISCUSSION: In the current era, the procedure of choice for simple transposition is the neonatal arterial switch operation. There are very few indications for an atrial-level switch in the neonate. Ventriculoarterial and atrioventricular discordance are the morphologic hallmarks of corrected transposition. In simple transposition, ventriculoarterial discordance and atrioventricular concordance are present. Cardiac catheterization is rarely if ever required in simple transposition. The arterial switch operation has a low rate of long-term complications and baffle obstruction is not an issue, as there is no baffle used in the arterial switch operation. Physiologically, simple transposition does present in the neonatal procedure with progressive cyanosis manifesting soon after birth and worsening with ductal closure.
Textbook: Page 1253 ANSWER: E

7. When comparing medical and surgical therapies for patients with chronic stable angina and three-vessel coronary disease, the patient group that benefits the most from coronary artery bypass grafting (CABG) in terms of survival and late cardiac events is characterized by:

A. Left ventricular ejection fraction (LVEF) greater than 50% and mild angina.
B. LVEF between 30 and 50% and moderate angina.
C. LVEF between 30 and 50% and severe angina.
D. LVEF less than 30% and severe angina.
E. LVEF greater than 50% and severe angina.

DISCUSSION: In comparisons of medical and surgical therapy outcomes, survival benefits appear most pronounced when CABG was performed in patients with the poorest left ventricular function combined with severe angina.
Textbook: Page 1272 ANSWER: D

8. When considering patients with chronic stable angina pectoris undergoing myocardial revascularization, the most powerful predictor of perioperative mortality is:

A. Age.
B. Sex.
C. Extensive coronary artery disease.
D. Number of prior myocardial infarctions.

E. Severity of left ventricular dysfunction.

DISCUSSION: The most powerful preoperative predictor of operative mortality, as well as long-term postoperative mortality, for patients with chronic stable angina pectoris having coronary artery bypass grafting is the degree of left ventricular dysfunction.

Textbook: Page 1278 ANSWER: E

9. Posterior postinfarction ventricular septal defect (VSD):

A. Has the same hospital mortality as anterior postinfarction VSD.
B. Often involves the posterior papillary muscles and requires mitral valve repair or replacement.
C. Rarely requires a patch for repair of the left ventricular free wall.
D. Is associated with fewer atrial ventricular conduction problems than anterior postinfarction VSD.
E. Usually involves infarction of the free wall of the right ventricle as well as the left ventricle.

DISCUSSION: Because the right coronary artery supplies the right ventricular as well as the left ventricular free wall, a posterior infarction often involves both right and left ventricular free walls.

Textbook: Page 1288 ANSWER: E

10. The use of the internal mammary artery as a conduit for myocardial revascularization in patients with chronic stable angina:

A. Increases the incidence of coronary reoperation.
B. Increases the risk of sternal wound problems.
C. Increases surgical mortality.
D. Improves long-term survival.

DISCUSSION: Both in-hospital and late survival are improved when the left internal mammary artery is grafted to the left anterior descending artery. Unilateral use of an internal mammary artery has not been associated with an increased risk of sternal infection in most large series.

Textbook: Page 1280 ANSWER: D

11. Re-do coronary artery bypass surgery is characterized by:

A. A lower incidence of postoperative myocardial infarction than in coronary artery bypass grafting (CABG) procedures.
B. Improved survival and freedom from angina in comparison with primary artery bypass surgery.
C. Mortality in the range of 3 to 10% that is almost exclusively the result of cardiac disease in contrast to primary CABG, in which mortality is most often the result of other organ system failure.
D. Reoperation that is always accomplished through a median sternotomy approach.

DISCUSSION: Although mortality in reoperative coronary artery bypass surgery has progressively improved, it still remains higher than that of primary CABG and is almost exclusively the result of cardiac causes in contrast to primary CABG.

Textbook: Page 1287 ANSWER: C

12. Which of the following is (are) indications for aortic valve replacement for aortic stenosis?

A. Syncope.
B. Congestive heart failure.
C. Angina.
D. Transvalvular gradient of 35 mm Hg without symptoms.

DISCUSSION: With progressive narrowing of the aortic valve area from the normal 3 to 4 cm^2 to 1 cm^2, patients become symptomatic. The classic symptoms produced by aortic stenosis are syncope, congestive heart failure, and angina. Once symptoms occur, life expectancy is limited to 2 to 5 years. Therefore, symptomatic aortic stenosis is an indication for aortic valve replacement. The risk of death with asymptomatic aortic stenosis is quite low, and aortic valve replacement is not indicated for asymptomatic patients with a transvalvular gradient less than 50 mm Hg.

Textbook: Page 1306 ANSWERS: A, B, C

13. Under which of the following circumstances may a patient logically be managed medically?

A. Moderate aortic insufficiency seen on echocardiography with normal left ventricular end-systolic dimensions.
B. Moderate to severe aortic insufficiency seen on echocardiography with cardiomegaly on chest roentgenogram.
C. Moderate aortic insufficiency seen on echocardiography with symptoms of congestive heart failure.
D. Moderate aortic insufficiency with an end-systolic left ventricular dimension of 70 mm as seen on echocardiography.

DISCUSSION: The left ventricle is usually able to compensate for the increased volume load imposed by aortic insufficiency for a long time. The natural history of asymptomatic aortic stenosis is excellent; 10-year survival for moderate aortic insufficiency managed medically is as high as 85 to 95%. Medical management typically consists of diuretics and afterload reduction. However, once the compensatory mechanisms begin to fail, survival is limited. Half of patients with signs and symptoms of congestive heart failure die within 2 years. Therefore, evidence of left ventricular dilation by echocardiography (left ventricular end-systolic dimension greater than 55 mm and cardiomegaly on chest x-ray) or symptoms of congestive heart failure are indications for aortic valve replacement.

Textbook: Page 1309 ANSWER: A

14. A patient with severe mitral regurgitation must undergo an emergent laparotomy for a perforated duodenal ulcer. Which of the following cardiac rhythms in the early postoperative period will most likely compromise the patient's overall hemodynamic condition?

A. Sinus rhythm at a rate of 60 beats/min.
B. Sinus rhythm at a rate of 100 beats/min.
C. Complete heart block with a ventricular rate of 60 beats/min.
D. Atrial fibrillation with a ventricular rate of 120 beats/min.

DISCUSSION: Because the incompetent mitral valve leaks during systole, the faster the heart rate (more systoles per minute), the greater the regurgitant volume. With tachycardia and increased regurgitant volume, the forward cardiac output decreases. Therefore, effective hemodynamic management of patients with mitral regurgitation includes control of the ventricular rate.

Textbook: Page 1302 ANSWER: D

15. A 40-year-old woman with evidence of left ventricular dysfunction suffers from severe mitral regurgitation secondary to mitral valve prolapse. At the time of mitral valve surgery, efforts should be made to:

A. Preserve the chordae tendineae.
B. Sever the chordae tendineae.
C. Place a bioprosthetic valve.
D. Examine the aortic valve for evidence of pathology.

DISCUSSION: The decision on whether the mitral valve may be repaired or replaced is finalized after direct inspection of the valve. Even if the valve must be replaced, chordae tendineae should be preserved. A mechanical advantage is afforded the left ventricle by the connection of its apex (by way of the papillary muscles) to the mitral annulus via the chordae tendineae; elimination of this connection by removal of the entire mitral apparatus leads to loss of left ventricular function. Preservation of at least some of the chordae tendineae at the time of mitral valve replacement results in much better long-term left ventricular function than mitral valve replacement with chordal separation.

Textbook: Page 1304 ANSWER: A

16. A 65-year-old asymptomatic man with known aortic stenosis is followed wtih annual Doppler echocardiography. Which of the following permits determination of aortic valve area?

A. The pressure half-time.
B. The Gorlin formula.
C. The continuity equation.
D. Planimetry of the valve.

DISCUSSION: The Gorlin formula uses information derived from cardiac catheterization. The pressure half-time is used to assess the severity of mitral stenosis. Planimetry of the valve does not permit calculation of the valve area. The Doppler echocardiogram does allow determination of the transaortic valve gradient, and use of the continuity equation permits calculation of the aortic valve area.

Textbook: Page 1305 ANSWER: C

NOTES

NOTES

CHAPTER 15

VASCULAR

1. Elective surgery for the asymptomatic patient is most often performed when aneurysm size is:

A. 2 to 3 cm.
B. 4 to 5 cm.
C. 5 to 6 cm.
D. 6 to 7 cm.

DISCUSSION: Aneurysm growth accelerates as size increases. The risk of rupture within 1 year for aneurysms smaller than 5 cm is 4%, but this risk increases to 43% at 6 cm or larger and to 80% at 8 cm or larger. Most frequently, patients with aneurysms 5 cm or larger are considered for elective surgery. However, patients with documented aneurysm enlargement or symptoms indicating aneurysm expansion are also considered candidates.
Textbook: Page 1314 ANSWER: C

2. The initial diagnostic test most frequently used to confirm the existence of a thoracic aneurysm is:

A. Aortography.
B. X-ray.
C. Transesophageal echocardiography.
D. Computed tomography (CT) scan.

DISCUSSION: All of the above diagnostic tools may be used at some point in patient treatment, but the CT scan has the best sensitivity and specificity, and lays the groundwork in aneurysm detection, providing superior overall definition of aneurysm size, location, and extent.
Textbook: Page 1315 ANSWER: D

3. In which segment of the aorta do aortic dissections most commonly originate?

A. Ascending aorta.
B. Aortic arch.
C. Thoracoabdominal aorta.
D. Abdominal aorta.

DISCUSSION: Sixty to 70 percent of aneurysm dissections occur in the anterior tubular portion of the ascending aorta.
Textbook: Page 1328 ANSWER: A

4. Which artery arises from an intercostal artery and plays a critical role in delivering blood to the spinal cord?

A. Vertebral artery.
B. Anterior spinal artery.
C. Posterior spinal artery.
D. Arteria radicularis magna.

DISCUSSION: The arteria radicularis magna, also known as the artery of Adamkiewicz, arises from an intercostal artery at the lower thoracic or upper lumbar level of the aorta with a branch to the anterior spinal artery below the spinal cord and another to anastomose with the ramus of the posterior spinal artery lying anterior to the dorsal roots. It is sometimes the main supply to the lower two thirds of the cord, making the reattachment of intercostal arteries in thoracoabdominal aortic repair of critical importance.
Textbook: Page 1323 ANSWER: D

5. In thoracoabdominal aortic repair, since the introduction of the protective adjuncts of distal aortic perfusion and cerebrospinal fluid drainage, which operative component is no longer a statistically significant risk factor?

A. Renal function.
B. Age.
C. Clamp time.
D. Aneurysm extent.

DISCUSSION: During the era of cross-clamp and go, all of the above were statistically significant risk factors in patient outcome. Distal aortic perfusion and cerebrospinal fluid drainage diminished the effects of both clamp time and aneurysm extent and eliminated the statistical significance of age as a risk factor.
Textbook: Page 1327 ANSWER: B

6. Vertebrobasilar system transient ischemic attacks are characterized by all of the following symptoms except:

A. Extremity numbness and weakness.
B. Diplopia.
C. Dysarthria.
D. Monocular visual loss.
E. Loss of balance.

DISCUSSION: Transient monocular visual loss or amaurosis fugax is characteristic of carotid-based embolic events. The ophthalmic artery is the first major branch of the internal carotid artery and the conduit through which thromboatherosclerotic emboli coming from the carotid bifurcation travel to the central retinal artery where transient obstruction causes monocular symptoms. Visual symptoms associated with vertebrobasilar insufficiency are characterized by bilateral visual symptoms, usually homonymous hemianopsia. All of the other symptoms can be caused by vertebrobasilar insufficiency.

Textbook: Page 1341 ANSWER: D

7. The strongest predictor of stroke in a patient presenting with hemispheric transient ischemic attacks is:

A. Severity of ipsilateral carotid stenosis.
B. Presence of hypercoagulable state.
C. Male sex.
D. Hypertension.
E. Inflammatory cells within the carotid plaque.

DISCUSSION: The data from the North American Symptomatic Carotid Endarterectomy Trial (NASCET) documented a strong positive correlation between risk of stroke and severity of carotid stenosis in symptomatic patients. The risk of stroke in patients treated with medical therapy for 2 years is 22% (50 to 69% stenosis), 21% (70 to 79% stenosis), 27% (80 to 89% stenosis), and 35% (90 to 99% stenosis). Based on epidemiologic data, male sex and hypertension are risk factors for stroke but are not strong prognostic indicators in individual patients. Hypercoagulable states can be associated with strokes, particularly in young patients presenting with symptoms, but are not strong predictors. Inflammatory cells within carotid plaques are pathologic changes that have been associated with plaque instability. It is not known whether these pathologic changes predispose to stroke.

Textbook: Page 1344 ANSWER: A

8. Carotid endarterectomy is most beneficial in a patient with a 70% carotid stenosis and transient symptoms of:

A. Diplopia.
B. Upper extremity numbness and weakness.
C. Confusion.
D. Dysarthria.
E. Monocular visual loss.

DISCUSSION: Diplopia is associated with vertebrobasilar distribution transient ischemic attacks (TIAs). Carotid endarterectomy would not be expected to alleviate this symptom. Confusion has multiple causes and is rarely associated with carotid artery occlusive disease. Dysarthria can be associated with carotid-based TIAs but is also associated with vertebrobasilar insufficiency. Monocular visual loss is a carotid-based symptom; however, it has a more benign natural history than hemispheric symptoms such as upper extremity numbness and weakness when treated with medical treatment alone. Therefore, the benefit of carotid endarterectomy is greater in the setting of hemispheric TIAs than in the setting of monocular visual symptoms.

Textbook: Page 1345 ANSWER: B

9. A stroke immediately following carotid endarterectomy is most likely due to:

A. Omission of perioperative aspirin.
B. Intracerebral hemorrhage.
C. Hypotension.
D. Lack of intraoperative shunting.
E. Carotid occlusion.

DISCUSSION: Of the choices, thrombotic carotid occlusion is the most likely to cause stroke immediately following carotid endarterectomy. Perioperative aspirin in low doses has been shown to modestly, but significantly, reduce the rate of adverse cardiovascular events (stroke, myocardial infarction, and death) after endarterectomy. However, lack of aspirin or other antiplatelet therapy has not been documented to cause stroke after endarterectomy. Intracerebral hemorrhage is a devastating but very uncommon cause of perioperative neurologic deficits. Hypotension has been anecdotally associated with postoperative stroke but causation has not been documented. The same is true of failure to use intraoperative shunting.

Textbook: Page 1348 ANSWER: E

10. Morbidity and mortality following carotid endarterectomy are highest among:

A. Neurosurgeons.
B. General surgeons.
C. Vascular surgeons.
D. Cardiothoracic surgeons.
E. Inexperienced surgeons.

DISCUSSION: The obvious answer here is inexperience of the surgeon. Many studies have documented that individual surgeon volume (regardless of training background) is an important determinant of outcomes. Surgeons performing low numbers of carotid endarterectomies (less than 5 to 10 annually) have higher rates of complications. Any surgeon performing this operation must have in-depth experience in the management of patients with cerebrovascular disease and the performance of carotid endarterectomy.

Textbook: Page 1350 ANSWER: E

11. The appropriate management of a 67-year-old woman who presents to the emergency department with a pulsatile abdominal mass, abdominal pain, and blood pressure of 80/40 is:

A. Emergency ultrasonography to confirm the presence of an abdominal aortic aneurysm.
B. Emergency computed tomography (CT) scan to assist in planning surgical treatment.
C. Immediate transport to the operating room for surgical exploration of the abdomen.
D. Initial resuscitation with intravenous fluids and reassessment.

DISCUSSION: Patients with ruptured aortic aneurysms require immediate surgical repair. If the patient is unstable and an abdominal aortic aneurysm has been previously diagnosed or a pulsatile abdominal mass is present, no further evaluation is performed and the patient is transferred to the operating room without additional tests. Stable patients with a questionable diagnosis may undergo CT, which can confirm the presence of an aneurysm as well as demonstrate its extent, the site of rupture, and the degree of iliac involvement. In patients without a pulsatile mass who are not stable enough to undergo CT, the presence of an aneurysm can be confirmed by bedside ultrasound. This does not demonstrate aortic rupture but will confirm the presence of an aortic aneurysm. Acutely expanding aneurysms may present with abdominal pain and tenderness on palpation. These are prone to rupture and should be repaired on an emergent basis.

Textbook: Page 1365 ANSWER: C

12. Which of the following statements regarding splenic artery aneurysms is true?

A. They are more common in men.
B. They should always be repaired even if small because of an unpredictable risk of rupture.
C. They are less common than hepatic artery aneurysms but more common than mesenteric artery aneurysms.
D. If discovered in a woman of childbearing age, elective aneurysm repair should be performed.

DISCUSSION: Visceral or splanchnic artery aneurysms are relatively uncommon but they are important to recognize and treat because roughly 25% present as emergencies and 8.5% result in death. Involved arteries and their relative frequencies include the splenic (60%), hepatic (20%), superior mesenteric (5.5%), and other arterial (each less than 5%). Splenic artery aneurysms occur most frequently in females with a female-to-male ratio of 4:1. This unusual sex predilection is likely related to acquired derangements of the arterial wall influenced by a number of processes including medial fibrodysplasia, portal hypertension, repeated pregnancy, penetrating or blunt abdominal trauma, pancreatitis, and infection. Women of childbearing age who have splenic artery aneurysms are at particularly high risk of death due to aneurysm rupture and should have elective repair. Symptomatic or ruptured aneurysms also warrant immediate repair. Surgical techniques for treating splenic artery aneurysms include simple proximal and distal ligation without arterial reconstruction for proximal aneurysms, and splenectomy versus aneurysm exclusion and vascular reconstruction for salvage of the spleen.

Textbook: Page 1371 ANSWER: D

13. Which of the following statements is true regarding endovascular abdominal aortic aneurysm repair?

A. This procedure is experimental and should not be recommended for routine clinical use.
B. Most patients can be evaluated preoperatively with ultrasonography alone.
C. Prolonged surveillance with periodic imaging is required postoperatively.
D. Endoleak refers to a contained aneurysm rupture after treatment with an endoluminal graft.

DISCUSSION: Endovascular aneurysm repair differs from open surgical repair in that the prosthetic graft is introduced into the aneurysm through the femoral arteries and fixed in place to the nonaneurysmal infrarenal neck and iliac arteries with self-expanding or balloon-expandable stents rather than sutures. A major abdominal incision is thus avoided and patient morbidity related to the procedure is much reduced. Candidates for this procedure include patients with a proximal infrarenal neck at least 1 to 2 cm in length and common iliac arteries for proximal and distal fixation of an endograft, without excessive tortuosity and with appropriate iliofemoral access. The benefits of this procedure are quicker recovery and lower morbidity, and it is often the best treatment option for high-risk patients. Extensive preoperative evaluation, including computed tomography or magnetic resonance angiographic imaging, is necessary to define the aneurysm morphology. Assessment of aneurysm length, diameter, angulation, relationship to renal arteries, and iliac artery tortuosity is important in patient selection. At this time there is no long-term follow-up, and the procedure should be undertaken with the understanding that prolonged surveillance with periodic imaging will be required and that reintervention may become necessary. Endovascular aneurysm repair is associated with a unique set of complications. Incomplete exclusion of the aneurysm sac with continued perfusion is referred to as endoleak and occurs in 9 to 44% of cases. Endoleaks related to the stent graft attachment sites may be associated with continued aneurysm expansion and risk of rupture. Such endoleaks can often be fixed by endovascular methods. Other complications include graft migration and stent graft occlusion.

Textbook: Page 1364 ANSWER: C

14. Approximately what percent of arterial emboli are cardiac in origin?

A. 15%.
B. 35%.
C. 55%.
D. 75%.

DISCUSSION: Over 75% of peripheral emboli are cardiogenic in origin. The most common predisposing factors are atrial fibrillation and emboli from mural embolus after a myocardial infarction. The source of cardiogenic emboli is best determined by clinical presentation and transesophageal echocardiography. Although rheumatic heart disease was formerly a common source of distal embolization, more recently prosthetic heart valves have become a more common source of distal embolization.

Textbook: Page 1384 ANSWER: D

15. Which of the following statements is false?

A. "Blue toe syndrome" is due to embolization of cholesterol crystals.
B. Blue toe syndrome often occurs after arterial catheterization.
C. Blue toe syndrome usually presents with

preservation of proximal pulses but absence of pedal pulses.
D. Blue toe syndrome is not treated with intra-arterial thrombolytic therapy.

DISCUSSION: Diffuse microembolization of cholesterol debris from the aorta and other proximal large vessels can result in "blue toe syndrome." This syndrome is characterized by bluish discoloration and ischemic lesions of the toes and heels in the setting of palpable proximal and distal pulses right down to the pedal level. There also may be changes of the livedo reticularis on the skin of the lower extremities. This syndrome most frequently occurs after intraluminal catheterization but may occur spontaneously. Given the nature of these microemboli, intra-arterial thrombolytic therapy has no role in the management of this problem.
Textbook: Page 1385 ANSWER: C

16. Which statement is true concerning claudication?
A. In severe cases it manifests as nocturnal calf pain.
B. Ultimately, 75 to 80% of patients require revascularization for limb salvage.
C. It is a marker for coronary artery disease and reduced survival.
D. Exercise and risk factor modifications are effective therapy for fewer than 25% of patients.

DISCUSSION: Arterial claudication is a marker for systemic atherosclerosis and coronary artery disease. Natural history studies reveal a mortality rate of approximately 5% per year for patients with claudication, with heart disease being the major cause of death. The majority (60% or more) of these patients do not progress to critical ischemia, particularly if they abstain from smoking and control other risk factors. With the addition of a structured exercise program, a significant percentage of patients improve their walking distance and the majority at least remain stable. True ischemic rest pain is localized to the foot and is often nocturnal; calf pain at rest is usually secondary to benign muscle cramps and is not a manifestation of arterial insufficiency.
Textbook: Page 1389 ANSWER: C

17. The most common cause of renovascular hypertension among patients less than 50 years of age is:
A. Abdominal aortic coarctation.
B. Medial fibroplasia.
C. Atherosclerosis.
D. Renal artery aneurysm.

DISCUSSION: Abdominal aortic coarctation is an extremely rare developmental anomaly that becomes evident with maturation among patients less than 30 years of age. Medial fibroplasia is by far the most common variety of fibromuscular dysplasia involving the renal artery. It is the most common cause of renovascular hypertension among children and adults less than 50 years of age, typically affecting women. Atherosclerosis involving the renal artery and adjacent aorta is the most common cause of renovascular hypertension, but it occurs in the older age group, among whom advanced atherosclerosis is most prevalent. Renal artery aneurysm is associated with hypertension in rare patients, some of whom have fibromuscular dysplasia.
Textbook: Page 1394 ANSWER: B

18. Among patients with atherosclerotic renovascular hypertension, kidney revascularization results in improvement or cure of hypertension in:
A. 25%.
B. 50%.
C. 75%.
D. 100%.

DISCUSSION: In the literature, definitions of benefit by cure or improvement of hypertension vary from report to report. Rigorous series define cure as average systolic pressure less than 150 and diastolic pressure less than 90 with the patient on no antihypertensive medications. Improvement after revascularization implies significant reduction of blood pressure on the same or fewer medications. The reported rates of cure range from 25 to 40% in the literature, with improvement ranging from 45 to 70%. Overall, combined cure and improvement rates are no less than 75% and range as high as 90%. Early results appear similar for surgical and percutaneous methods of revascularization.
Textbook: Page 1398 ANSWER: C

19. Diagnosis of acute mesenteric ischemia is most likely when the patient has:
A. Elevation of the white blood cell (WBC) count.
B. Diffuse pain out of proportion to tenderness.
C. Gas in the cecum on kidneys, ureters, and bladder (KUB) series.
D. Bloody stool in the rectum.

DISCUSSION: Elevation of the WBC count occurs as part of the inflammatory response to infection, ischemia, and necrosis. It is nonspecific, occurring in many abdominal conditions. The symptom of severe diffuse pain with disproportionately mild or moderate signs of abdominal tenderness is a classic presentation in the early stages of mesenteric ischemia. Reduced blood flow to the viscera creates pain without convincing signs of peritoneal irritation until the parietal peritoneum becomes involved during later stages when transmural bowel damage has developed. Gas in the cecum is nonspecific and quite normal as an isolated finding on KUB. Colonic distention as evidenced by an abnormal gas pattern on KUB may be pathologic and associated with mesenteric ischemia, among other illnesses. Although bloody stool in the rectum may occur with mucosal injury caused by acute mesenteric ischemia, this sign is nonspecific and occurs typically with more common sources of gastrointestinal hemorrhage.
Textbook: Page 1399 ANSWER: B

20. The most prominent risk factor for nonocclusive mesenteric ischemia is:

A. Use of digoxin.
B. Hypercoagulable state.
C. Prolonged hemodynamic collapse.
D. Atrial fibrillation.

DISCUSSION: Nonocclusive mesenteric ischemia is caused by vasoconstriction after hemodynamic collapse among some patients with severe congestive heart failure, cardiogenic shock, sepsis, or hemorrhage. The clinical association between digoxin and nonocclusive mesenteric ischemia is explained by wide use of digitalis preparations in years past in patients with cardiac disease and increased intestinal arterial resistance caused by digitalis under circumstances of portal venous congestion. This association is much less prominent in recent years with the diminishing use of digitalis preparations. Hypercoagulable states are classically associated with mesenteric venous occlusion, not nonocclusive mesenteric arterial ischemia. Atrial fibrillation is a risk factor for acute embolic occlusion of the mesenteric vasculature.

Textbook: Page 1400 ANSWER: C

21. Which of the following is most predictive for successful healing of a simple (transphalangeal) toe amputation in a diabetic patient presenting with a small ulceration at the tip of the second toe?

A. Presence of a palpable popliteal pulse.
B. No prior symptoms of claudication or rest pain.
C. Doppler occlusion pressure at the ipsilateral ankle of 240 mm Hg.
D. Toe pressure of 42 mm Hg.

DISCUSSION: Peripheral arterial disease in diabetic patients has distinctive anatomic characteristics, including a propensity for the infrapopliteal vessels and a diffuse medial calcinosis of the muscular arteries in the lower leg. It is not uncommon to find a normal popliteal pulse and falsely elevated ankle occlusion pressures in a diabetic patient with critical forefoot ischemia. If the disease is localized to the calf with relative sparing of the superficial femoral artery, often there may be no prior symptoms of claudication prior to the onset of tissue necrosis. Because the calcification rarely extends to the digital level, toe pressures retain some clinical value in predicting healing, particularly if they are higher than 40 mm Hg.

Textbook: Page 1376 ANSWER: D

22. Which of the following statements is incorrect?

A. Takayasu's arteritis predominantly affects the muscular arteries in middle-aged women of Asian descent.
B. The primary treatment for Buerger's disease is smoking cessation.
C. Giant cell arteritis should be suspected in a 50-year-old patient with arm claudication and headaches.
D. Raynaud's disease is most successfully managed by sympathectomy.

DISCUSSION: Takayasu's arteritis primarily affects the aorta and its major trunks (elastic vessels), with a predilection for younger women. The overwhelming majority of patients with Buerger's disease are dramatically improved by abstinence from smoking. Headaches (superficial temporal artery) and arm claudication (major aortic arch trunks) should prompt consideration of giant cell arteritis, particularly with other constitutional symptoms or signs (elevated erythrocyte sedimentation rate). Primary therapy for Raynaud's disease focuses on avoidance of triggers, calcium channel blockade, and sympatholytic drugs.

Textbook: Page 1375 ANSWER: A

23. Which of the following statement is true concerning the risks and preparation for patients undergoing contrast angiography?

A. Patients with a history of prior major allergic reactions to conventional contrast can be offered nonionic contrast media with minimal risk of recurrence.
B. A postcatheterization femoral pseudoaneurysm in a patient requiring urgent coronary artery bypass grafting (CABG) is best managed by ultrasound-guided compression en route to the operating room.
C. Preparation of a diabetic patient with a serum creatinine of 2 mg per 100 ml for contrast arteriography requires strict fluid restriction before and after dye injection to avoid volume overload.
D. Percutaneous angioplasty (with or without stenting) is the initial treatment of choice for most patients with isolated common iliac disease.

DISCUSSION: Although the overall incidence of allergic reactions appears to be less with nonionic media, patients with a prior major reaction remain at elevated risk regardless of the agent employed and must be premedicated and closely monitored if contrast exposure cannot be avoided. A femoral pseudoaneurysm in a patient undergoing urgent CABG, with the attendant need for high-dose heparinization, is best managed by direct surgical repair as a simultaneous procedure. Diabetic patients with renal insufficiency are at a high risk for contrast nephropathy, particularly if they are hypovolemic; careful volume loading before and after contrast injection is critical to avoid renal failure. Short- and long-term results of percutaneous angioplasty for favorable (short stenoses) lesions of the common iliac artery are excellent, making this the initial treatment of choice in suitable candidates.

Textbook: Page 1350 ANSWER: D

24. The most urgent concern in a patient with penetrating cervical vascular trauma is:

A. Imminent hemispheric neurologic deficit.

B. Loss of airway.
C. An associated thoracic injury.
D. Hemorrhagic shock.

DISCUSSION: Loss of an airway is always a major and urgent concern. In a patient with a cervical vascular injury, a large, expanding hematoma can jeopardize the airway very quickly. The deep cervical fascia that encircles the trachea also contains the carotid artery and internal jugular vein. An expanding hematoma in this contained fascial compartment can impinge on the trachea, causing considerable deviation very quickly. In an emergency center, the surgeon might be faced with a consideration for an urgent surgical airway. If there is a large contained (arterial) hematoma surrounding the trachea, this hematoma is released at the time of the incision of the deep cervical fascia, often with catastrophic results. Early oral tracheal or nasotracheal intubation is the preferred treatment under these circumstances.

Textbook: Page 1405 ANSWER: B

25. A 25-year-old patient sustains a gunshot injury to the abdomen. On exploration, he has a large central retroperitoneal hematoma above the transverse mesocolon. The best surgical approach would be:

A. Do not explore if the hematoma is not expanding.
B. Proximal aortic control at the diaphragm and medial rotation of the left-sided viscera.
C. Immediate direct approach through the lesser omentum.
D. Proximal aortic control at the diaphragm and direct approach through the lesser omentum.

DISCUSSION: Patients with retroperitoneal hematomas are among the most challenging problems faced by any surgeon at any time. Such hematomas may be upper midline, lower midline, pelvic, or lateral; however, the upper midline hematomas are the toughest of the tough challenges. It is imperative that such hematomas be explored, but ONLY after proximal and distal control is achieved, if time allows. A surgeon should never just plunge into the middle of such a hematoma. With a rotation of the viscera to the right, beginning lateral to the left colon, and going behind the kidney, on top of the psoas muscle, a relatively clean plane free from hematoma is found. The first assistant can control aortic pressure by digitally holding the aorta at the diaphragm. Survival is not enhanced by opening the chest first for proximal control. A vascular clamp may be placed easily on either side of the aortic injury and an orderly reconstruction performed. Dissection anterior to the kidney or through the lesser sac causes the surgeon to encounter dense fibrous and nervous tissue, making dissection almost impossible.

Textbook: Page 1410 ANSWER: B

26. A 70-year-old woman is brought to the emergency center after having sustained multiple injuries in a motor vehicle accident. Her injuries include diffuse axonal injury of the brain, severe bilateral lung contusions, an intraparenchymal liver hematoma, and a fractured left femur. Aortography reveals a blunt injury to the descending aorta with a mediastinal hematoma. She is hemodynamically stable. The safest course of action at this time is:

A. Immediate thoracotomy to repair the life-threatening aortic injury using a direct clamp repair.
B. Observation in the intensive care unit with close monitoring and pharmacologic control of the blood pressure.
C. Thoracotomy and aortic repair using a pump-assisted atriofemoral bypass.
D. Thoracotomy within 6 hours of injury because the risk of free rupture quadruples after this time frame.

DISCUSSION: Patients more than 55 years of age have a significantly increased mortality (for similarly staged aortic blunt injury) compared with a "younger" patient counterpart. In any patient, especially an older one, multiple injuries also cause problems of prioritization and timing. Any patient with an aortic injury who is hemodynamically stable for the first 4 to 6 hours after a blunt trauma rarely dies of an aortic rupture–related death, if the blood pressure is pharmacologically kept lower than preinjury blood pressure. Deaths in this group are most often due to head injury or multisystem injury. In an elderly patient with multiple injuries who is hemodynamically stable, the patient is well served by altering the shear forces on the aortic wall by pharmacologic means and delaying surgery for hours, days, weeks, or even months, until the other injuries have been addressed. Even then, there is increasing consideration for endovascular stented graphs in patients with chronic, post-traumatic thoracic false aneurysms.

Textbook: Page 1407 ANSWER: B

27. Regarding the use of grafts in vascular trauma, which of the following statements is correct?

A. The saphenous vein is the graft material of choice for a contaminated operative field.
B. The failure mode of synthetic grafts in an infected field is the same as vein grafts.
C. Vein is the graft material of choice in upper extremity and below-knee reconstructions.
D. Polytetrafluoroethylene (PTFE) grafts have excellent long-term patency when used for venous reconstructions.

DISCUSSION: Much debate exists regarding the use of substitute conduits in vascular trauma; however, much of this debate and bias is not based on scientifically supportive data. More than 50 laboratory studies have been reported citing (in the experimental animal) that in a contaminated wound, the incidence of complications is identical whether autogenous or synthetic material is used as a substitute conduit. Complications in the experimental animal and in human clinical studies are different, however. Complica-

tions in association with a substitute autogenous conduit are usually graft dissolution and hemorrhage, often in very inopportune times and places and often with an accompanying death. On the other hand, an infection surrounding a synthetic conduit may result in sepsis, suture line aneurysm, distal embolization, or thrombosis. These later complications are usually easier to manage than those surrounding autogenous tissue. There is further evidence that when acutely moved from its vasa vasorum connections, the saphenous vein is a dead collagen tube for the first several weeks after scavenge and insertion in a second site. Ultimately fibroblasts and an endothelium can be demonstrated, but viable cells cannot be demonstrated acutely. Thus the scavenged saphenous vein is acutely a dead collagen tube and subject to collagenase activity of the bacteria. On the other hand, when dealing with vessels less than 5 mm in diameter, it is preferable to use a saphenous vein from the patient, as the thrombosis rate of synthetic material less than 5 mm is high. The exact thrombosis rate of *any* conduit placed for posttraumatic venous reconstruction is unknown.
Textbook: Page 1414 ANSWER: C

28. In a patient with gunshot injury to the lower abdomen involving the sigmoid and the left common iliac artery, the best reconstructive option in the presence of significant spillage is:

A. Colon repair, closure of the abdomen, and a femorofemoral bypass.
B. Sigmoid colostomy and repair of the artery with PTFE graft.
C. Sigmoid repair and an obturator foramen bypass.
D. Sigmoid repair, tie-off of the common iliac artery, and four-compartment fasciotomy.

DISCUSSION: It is most preferable to avoid problems of vascular conduit infection, just as it is important to prevent other postinjury complications. An occasional patient can tolerate the acute ligation of a common iliac artery, but might develop a calf compartment syndrome. It is imperative that a lateral lower abdominal hematoma be explored and the injury be either ligated or reconstructed. Primary closure of colon injuries can be accomplished at least 70 to 80% of the time, and the abdominal contamination can be lavaged clear relatively quickly. PTFE grafts can be easily and quickly inserted into an area of common iliac artery injury, and PTFE has relative resistance to infection. If a perigraft infection occurs in the patient described, the graft can then be removed, even through an extraperitoneal approach, and the common iliac artery ligated after removal of the PTFE. In that instance, at a delayed time and if necessary, a femorofemoral artery crossover graft can be performed.
Textbook: Page 1411 ANSWER: B

29. The calf pressure that should cause the surgeon to do a fasciotomy is:

A. 10 cm H_2O.
B. 20 cm H_2O.
C. 30 cm H_2O.
D. 40 cm H_2O.
E. 50 cm H_2O.

DISCUSSION: The figure of 30 cm H_2O is most often cited as the absolute number at which decompression of the area is required. In a hypotensive patient, or one who has excessive venous pressure, the relative index at which decompression might be required could be lower. Measurement of compartment pressures may be accomplished using a variety of devices. Under investigation and a subject of numerous recent reports is the use of machines that use near infrared spectroscopy to measure oxygen consumption in muscle compartments as a guide to the timing of fasciotomy. Such studies have inconsistently correlated their findings with compartment pressures.
Textbook: Page 1414 ANSWER: C

30. Which of the following questions regarding venous anatomy and/or physiology is true?

A. Relative to the foot, venous valves are most abundant in the proximal lower extremity, and the number of valves increases as one moves toward the central venous circulation.
B. Venous valves are composed of bicuspid leaflets of connective tissue covered by endothelium, and a reverse flow velocity of at least 30 cm/sec is required for venous valve closure.
C. The lesser saphenous vein ascends in the posterior midline of the lower leg to pierce the deep fascia and join with the peroneal vein in the proximal calf.
D. The venous system contains approximately one half of the blood volume in the resting state, and approximately 150 ml of blood is shifted to the legs on assumption of the upright position.
E. Calf muscle contraction generates venous pressures of approximately 75 mm Hg, and the calf muscle contraction impedes arterial perfusion by increasing venous pressure.

DISCUSSION: Venous valves are composed of bicuspid leaflets of connective tissue covered by endothelium. The normal valve sinus is wider than the adjacent normal vein segment, and therefore one observes vein dilation at the level of a venous valve. The open valve cusps do not lay flat against the vein wall and are engaged by the retrograde flow of blood. A reverse flow velocity of at least 30 cm/sec is required for venous valve closure.
Textbook: Page 1418 ANSWER: B

31. When evaluating a patient for suspected acute deep vein thrombosis (DVT), which of the following statements regarding diagnosis is accurate?

A. Clinical features are not helpful in evaluating patients with suspected DVT.
B. Noninvasive studies such as impedance plethysmography and phleborrheography are

as effective as venous duplex imaging for the initial screening of patients for acute DVT.
C. Magnetic resonance venography (MRV) is costly, not usually available for routine venous diagnostic studies, and metallic implants and claustrophobia limit its application. However, the true value of MRV is likely to be in those patients with calf vein thrombosis.
D. Of the blood tests investigated to assist with the diagnosis of acute DVT, the D-dimer level has been found to be helpful. A negative D-dimer test in patients with suspected DVT has a high negative predictive value.
E. Radioisotope testing for DVT is increasing in popularity and will likely be helpful in patients with first-time DVT.

DISCUSSION: During the past two decades, the use of blood tests has been investigated to assist with the diagnosis of acute DVT. A large number of blood studies have been evaluated, and the D-dimer test has been shown to be the most useful. Although D-dimer levels are elevated in postoperative and acutely ill patients, a negative D-dimer test in patients with suspected DVT has a high negative predictive value, and can be used to exclude proximal DVT in these patients.
Textbook: Page 1424 ANSWER: D

32. Which of the following statements regarding the natural history of acute deep vein thrombosis (DVT) is true?

A. The long-term complication of acute DVT (the postthrombotic syndrome) is unavoidable.
B. The pathophysiology of the postthrombotic syndrome is ambulatory venous hypertension, with the two main components being valvular incompetence and venous obstruction.
C. Maximal venous outflow methods are reliable measures of the degree of chronic venous obstruction.
D. Residual venous obstruction is protective against severe ambulatory venous hypertension in patients with valvular incompetence.
E. Patients who undergo spontaneous lysis of their acute DVT and patients with persisting obstruction have essentially equivalent chances of developing the postthrombotic syndrome.

DISCUSSION: The underlying pathophysiology of the postthrombotic syndrome is ambulatory venous hypertension contributed by the two components of residual venous obstruction and valvular incompetence.
Textbook: Page 1425 ANSWER: B

33. Low-molecular-weight heparin has been shown to be at least equivalent if not superior to unfractionated heparin in the treatment of patients with infrainguinal deep vein thrombosis (DVT). The reported advantages of low-molecular-weight heparin over unfractionated heparin include all of the following except:

A. Significantly improved bioavailability following subcutaneous injection.
B. Patients can be treated as outpatients without blood tests for monitoring anticoagulant level.
C. There is a more effective partial thromboplastin time (PTT) response per unit volume injected.
D. Although heparin-induced thrombocytopenia can occur with low-molecular-weight heparin compounds, its risk is reduced to approximately one seventh of unfractionated heparin.
E. There is less protein binding with low-molecular-weight compounds, and therefore less likelihood of heparin resistance.

DISCUSSION: Low-molecular-weight heparin compounds are assuming increasing importance in the treatment of acute venous thromboembolic disorders. They have significantly improved bioavailability after subcutaneous injection compared with unfractionated heparin, with 80 to 90% of the low-molecular-weight heparin injected subcutaneously reaching the bloodstream compared with 20% of unfractionated heparin. This improved bioavailability has allowed outpatient therapy of acute DVT, since intravenous injection is no longer required. Because low-molecular-weight heparins do not have any effect on the PTT, blood tests to monitor anticoagulation are not required. Prospective trials have shown a significant reduction in the incidence of heparin-induced thrombocytopenia, along with the associated reduction in thrombotic complications, to approximately one seventh that of unfractionated heparin. Unfractionated heparin is bound by circulation proteins, and occasionally heparin resistance is encountered as a result of this phenomenon. Low-molecular-weight heparins do not bind to circulating proteins; therefore heparin resistance is not encountered with these agents.
Textbook: Page 1427 ANSWER: C

34. Which of the following statements about lymphatic capillaries is (are) true?

A. These vessels have delicate tricuspid valves every 2 to 3 mm.
B. Lymphatic capillaries are less permeable than blood capillaries.
C. Lymphatic capillaries are more permeable than blood capillaries.
D. Lymphatic capillaries contain gaps large enough to admit particles as large as lymphocytes.

DISCUSSION: The transporting lymphatic vessels have valves but not lymphatic capillaries. The lymphatic capillaries accept particles including bacteria, red blood cells, and lymphocytes and transport them to regional lymph nodes.
Textbook: Page 1446 ANSWER: D

35. The following forces promote the formation of interstitial fluid except:

A. Increase in venous pressure.

B. Constrictive pericarditis.
C. Hypernatremia.
D. Hypoproteinemia.

DISCUSSION: Interstitial fluid production is a function of the hydrostatic and colloid osmotic pressures across the capillary membrane. Forces tending to increase interstitial fluid flux across the capillary membrane include obstruction to outflow of the capillary due to structural or functional obstruction in the venous system or increase in venous pressure from any cause, reduction in osmotic pressure due to hypoproteinemia, and increase in pore size due to local mediators of inflammation.
Textbook: Page 1446 ANSWER: C

36. The most frequent cause of primary lymphedema is:
A. A deficiency of transporting lymphatic channels.
B. Valvular incompetence in lymphatic channels.
C. Obstruction or removal of regional lymph nodes.
D. Thrombosis of lymphatic channels.

DISCUSSION: Primary lymphedema is most frequently due to hypoplasia or aplasia of extremity transporting lymphatic channels.
Textbook: Page 1448 ANSWER: A

37. Most patients with lymphedema can be managed by:
A. Pedicle transfer of lymphatic-bearing tissue into the affected area.
B. The use of elevation, elastic support garments, and massage therapy or mechanical pneumatic compression.
C. Lymphatic bypass using an autogenous vein graft.
D. Excision of hypertrophied, scarred fibrotic skin and subcutaneous tissue down to muscle fascia and coverage with split-thickness skin grafts.

DISCUSSION: The vast majority of patients with mild to moderate lymphedema can be managed with leg elevation, the use of elastic support garments, and some require mechanical pneumatic compression or massage therapy. Only patients with severe deforming elephantiasis require operative therapy.
Textbook: Page 1449 ANSWER: B

38. Which of the following statements is true concerning lymphangiomas?
A. Most lesions appear during the time of puberty.
B. These lesions are frequently responsive to low doses of radiation therapy.
C. The lesions usually grow slowly but may infiltrate local tissues.
D. Malignant transformation is frequent.

DISCUSSION: Lymphangiomas are congenital malformations of the lymphatic vessels. Most of these lesions appear at birth or during early infancy. The lesions grow slowly and infiltrate local tissues, but actual malignant degeneration is exceedingly rare. The lesions are not responsive to radiation therapy.
Textbook: Page 1451 ANSWER: C

39. For acute long-term dialysis the best option is:
A. Scribner shunt.
B. Bilateral femoral catheters.
C. Inferior vena caval catheter.
D. Internal jugular PermCath catheter.
E. Subclavian PermCath catheter.

DISCUSSION: The Scribner shunt is rarely used today. It destroys the potential for a natural fistula at the wrist and can become easily infected. Femoral catheters are used for acute dialysis but must be removed within days to prevent infection. A subclavian catheter can be used; however, the risk of subclavian stenosis is very high and it is not the first choice, although it may be necessary in some cases. An inferior vena caval line is a last resort in patients who have no other means of access. The best option is an internal jugular PermCath catheter. This causes the least amount of stenosis and gives immediate access for dialysis and can be used in some cases as long as a year.
Textbook: Page 1453 ANSWER: D

40. All of the following are appropriate steps in evaluating a patient for placement of a permanent vascular access except:
A. Check for the presence of a cephalic vein at the wrist and in the upper arm.
B. Perform an Allen test.
C. Do a venogram of arm veins.
D. In a patient with a history of home total parenteral nutrition, administer a subclavian venogram.
E. Perform a duplex study of arm veins.

DISCUSSION: All of the maneuvers are appropriate when evaluating a patient for placement of a permanent access except a venogram of arm veins. This does not give adequate information about the size and dynamics of veins. A duplex examination will do so and is the preferred method. A duplex examination can also determine whether a basilic vein transposition is possible. Evaluation of veins in the forearm and upper arm is appropriate to determine whether a natural fistula can be placed. The Allen test determines the adequacy of the palmar arch for placement of a wrist fistula. If a patient has had a history of a subclavian line at any time, a subclavian venogram rules out the possibility of subclavian stenosis or occlusion. Both stenosis and occlusion prevent successful placement of a permanent access.
Textbook: Page 1455 ANSWER: C

41. The most common complication after placement of a PTFE graft for dialysis is:
A. Arterial stenosis secondary to intimal hyperplasia.

B. Aneurysm blowout.
C. Venous stenosis secondary to intimal hyperplasia.
D. Infection.
E. Steal syndrome.

DISCUSSION: Aneurysm blowouts rarely occur today. There are occasional false aneurysms at the anastomotic line that can become problematic but do not truly blow out. The most common complication is venous stenosis caused by intimal hyperplasia. In a clotted graft this is the cause in over 90% of the cases. Arterial stenosis rarely occurs. Infection is the next most common complication after venous hyperplasia. It frequently results in removal of the graft. Steal syndrome occurs rarely but occurs more commonly in small women who are diabetic and more than 65 years of age.

Textbook: Page 1457 ANSWER: C

42. In a clotted arteriovenous Gore-Tex graft, arguments for surgery versus radiologic intervention include:

A. Patency is not as good in surgery.
B. The graft has a longer functional life in surgical intervention.
C. A temporary access can be averted in surgical intervention.
D. Patencies over 40% at 1 year are possible with surgical intervention.

DISCUSSION: There is a longer patency with surgical intervention compared with radiologic intervention. However, these patencies are rarely larger than 40% at 6 months. Marston and coworkers (1997) showed that surgery resulted in longer patency, that some lesions could not be attacked radiologically, and that surgery was required. Occasionally, temporary access is required in surgery.

Textbook: Page 1458 ANSWER: B

43. Peritoneal dialysis is useful in all of the following settings except:

A. Patients who are diabetic.
B. Patients who have ileus.
C. Patients who have a diaphragmatic hernia.
D. Patients who have a ventral hernia.

DISCUSSION: Peritoneal dialysis is useful in diabetics and gives smooth insulin control because insulin can be added to the dialysate. It is also useful in patients who have bleeding disorders and those who want control of their dialysis routine. Peritoneal dialysis catheter placement can cause ileus but this rarely lasts long enough to give permanent disability. Patients do have constipation with peritoneal dialysis. Patients with ventral hernias can undergo dialysis but may have to have the hernia repaired. Those patients with a diaphragmatic hernia cannot be dialyzed using peritoneal dialysis because of pulmonary compromise.

Textbook: Page 1459 ANSWER: C

NOTES

NOTES

CHAPTER 16

PEDIATRICS

1. Polyhydramnios is frequently observed in all of the following conditions except:

A. Esophageal atresia.
B. Duodenal atresia.
C. Pyloric atresia.
D. Hirschsprung's disease.
E. Congenital diaphragmatic hernia.

DISCUSSION: Polyhydramnios is defined as excessive amounts of fluid (more than 2000 ml) in the amniotic sac during pregnancy. The amniotic pool is a dynamic pool with a relatively rapid turnover. In the fourth intrauterine month the fetus begins to swallow amniotic fluid (25 to 40% of the volume) and absorbs the fluid from the upper gastrointestinal tract. The fluid is urinated back out into the amniotic pool by the fetal kidneys and a functioning bladder. Although there are maternal causes of polyhydramnios (cardiac failure, renal failure, other causes of fluid retention) and some idiopathic cases, many instances are related to the presence of fetal anomalies. These include central nervous system problems such as anencephaly, which prevents normal swallowing, and any high alimentary tract obstruction that blocks the passage of the amniotic fluid and prevents its absorption (including esophageal atresia, pyloric atresia, and duodenal atresia). In addition, infants with congenital diaphragmatic hernia have obstruction due to herniation of the stomach and bowel into the thoracic cavity. This is a poor prognostic finding in these infants. Hirschsprung's disease is a form of low intestinal obstruction, and therefore an adequate length of proximal patent intestine is available for absorption of the swallowed amniotic fluid and polyhydramnios is usually not present.

Textbook: Page 1466 ANSWER: D

2. Which of the following statements about Hirschsprung's disease is not true?

A. There are no ganglion cells seen in Auerbach plexus.
B. There is an increased incidence of Down's syndrome.
C. It is more common in girls.
D. It may be associated with enterocolitis.
E. It may involve the small intestine.

DISCUSSION: The affected segment of bowel in patients with Hirschsprung's disease has hypertrophic nerves in Auerbach intermyenteric plexus but no ganglion cells are present. Ganglion cells are also absent in Meissner submucosal plexus. Three to 5% of babies with Hirschsprung's disease also have Down's syndrome. Hirschsprung's disease should be suspected in infants with Down's syndrome who manifest evidence of abdominal distention and constipation. Hirschsprung's disease is much more common in boys (4:1). The enterocolitis of Hirschsprung's disease is a condition associated with delay in diagnosis, low bowel obstruction, severe abdominal distention, explosive diarrhea, and colonic mucosal ulceration. The course may be fulminant. This complication is associated with increased morbidity and mortality. Bacterial translocation and endotoxemia may complicate the condition. Treatment includes nasogastric suction, intravenous fluids, antibiotics, and rectal tube decompression of the obstructed rectosigmoid segment. In approximately 10% of cases, aganglionosis extends into varying lengths of small bowel. In rare instances, the entire small bowel and colon may be aganglionic.

Textbook: Page 1473 ANSWER: C

3. In infants with gastroschisis, which of the following statements is not true?

A. It is associated with malrotation.
B. There is a high incidence of associated anomalies.
C. There is prolonged adynamic ileus following repair.
D. It is complicated by intestinal atresia in 10 to 12% of cases.
E. It is not associated with chromosomal syndromes.

DISCUSSION: Because of intrauterine herniation of bowel to an extra-abdominal location, normal intestinal rotation and fixation do not occur. Most infants with gastroschisis have nonrotation. In contrast to infants with omphalocele, in which a high incidence of associated anomalies coexist, babies with gastroschisis have little else wrong. Following repair of the abdominal wall defect, infants with gastroschisis have a long delay in return of intestinal function. They usually require total parenteral nutrition to supply adequate caloric intake until gut function returns (3 to 4 weeks). Intestinal atresia is observed in 10 to 12% of neonates with gastroschisis. This is caused by bowel ischemia due to intrauterine volvulus or compression of the herniated viscera in a small, tight defect in the abdominal wall. Although infants with omphalocele frequently have chromosomal syn-

dromes such as Beckwith's syndrome or trisomy 13 to 15 or 16 to 18, babies with gastroschisis do not.
Textbook: Page 1479 ANSWER: B

4. In neonates with congenital diaphragmatic hernia, which of the following statements is true?

A. The defect is more common on the right side.
B. Survival is significantly improved by administration of pulmonary vasodilators.
C. An oxygen index of 20 is an indication for extracorporeal membrane oxygenation (ECMO).
D. Oligohydramnios is a frequent occurrence.
E. Mortality is the result of pulmonary hypoplasia.

DISCUSSION: In infants with congenital diaphragmatic hernia the defect is more common on the left side (85%). Polyhydramnios is sometimes noticed and is a poor prognostic indicator of survival. Oligohydramnios is noted in fetuses with urinary tract obstruction and may be associated with pulmonary hypoplasia with an intact diaphragm. Although pulmonary vasodilators were used extensively in babies with congenital diaphragmatic hernia, they have not significantly improved survival. An oxygen index of more than 40 is the usual indication for ECMO. Pulmonary hypoplasia is the main cause of mortality in babies with congenital diaphragmatic hernia.
Textbook: Page 1481 ANSWER: E

5. Which of the following statements is not true regarding the premature neonate?

A. A 15 to 20% right-to-left shunt occurs across the foramen ovale and patent ductus arteriosus.
B. Surfactant levels are normal after 34 weeks' gestation.
C. Fluid requirements are higher than in a full-term baby.
D. Rectal temperature is the best indicator of core body temperature.
E. Premature infants are more at risk for infection than full-term infants.

DISCUSSION: The newborn infant has a relatively elevated pulmonary artery pressure and shunts a significant amount of unoxygenated blood through the foramen ovale and patent ductus arteriosus. The normal PaO_2 below the ductus as measured through an umbilical artery catheter would be between 60 and 80 mm Hg. Surfactant levels do not approach normal until after the thirty-fourth week of gestation when enzyme levels in the surfactant pathway mature. Amniocentesis is performed to measure the lecithin-sphingomyelin ratio (L:S ratio) and determine whether maturation has occurred. Fluid requirements in the premature infant are between 140 and 150 ml per kg per day in comparison with the normal neonate in whom 80 ml per kg per day would be adequate. Increased insensible losses and the need for overhead warmers play a role in this increase. Axillary or skin probe temperature monitoring is more accurate than the rectal temperature in the neonate. The rectal temperature is not a good indicator of core body temperature until approximately 18 months of age. Premature infants lack immunoglobulin (Ig) A and have low levels of IgM, the C3b component of complement, and decreased opsonins. In addition, the white blood corpuscles have reduced phagocytic ability, creating an increased risk of infection. *Escherichia coli* and beta-hemolytic streptococcus are the two most common infectious agents affecting the neonate.
Textbook: Pages 1464–1465 ANSWER: D

6. In neonates with necrotizing enterocolitis, which of the following findings is an indication of significant bowel ischemia?

A. Increased gastric residuals.
B. Septic shock.
C. Cardiac failure due to a patent ductus arteriosus (PDA).
D. Elevated platelet count.
E. Erythema of the abdominal wall.

DISCUSSION: Necrotizing enterocolitis (NEC) is a condition that occurs in 2% of babies admitted to neonatal intensive care facilities. Increased gastric residuals can occur for a number of reasons, and are seen as an early indicator of NEC, but may not reflect the presence of ischemic bowel. Septic shock may be due to a wide variety of causes besides NEC. Cardiac failure due to PDA may predispose to NEC but is not necessarily an indicator of ischemic bowel. Most babies with NEC have a progressive decrease in their platelet count in association with bowel ischemia. Erythema of the abdominal wall is an indication for surgical exploration and is consistent with NEC with perforation and inflammation of the peritoneum and abdominal wall.
Textbook: Page 1476 ANSWER: E

7. The treatment of choice for neonates with uncomplicated meconium ileus is:

A. Observation.
B. Emergency laparotomy, bowel resection, and Bishop-Koop enterostomy.
C. Intravenous hydration and a Gastrografin enema.
D. Emergency laparotomy, bowel resection, and anastomosis.
E. Sweat chloride test and pancreatic enzyme therapy.

DISCUSSION: Meconium ileus is a form of intestinal obstruction that occurs in 10 to 15% of neonates with cystic fibrosis. The obstruction is related to intraluminal concretions of abnormal meconium. The treatment of choice is adequate hydration and evacuation with a hypertonic Gastrografin enema. The hyperosmolar contrast material causes an outpouring of fluids into the bowel lumen, which flushes out the obstructing meconium and negates the need for laparotomy. Observation alone is not a useful method of treatment.

When Gastrografin evacuation fails, laparotomy, placement of a pursestring suture in the bowel wall, and intraluminal irrigation with saline and Gastrografin (administered through a catheter inserted through a small enterotomy within the pursestring) often clears the obstructing meconium. This obviates the need for resection or enterostomy in most cases. Postoperatively, a sweat chloride test should be obtained to confirm the diagnosis of cystic fibrosis. Pancreatic enzyme should be given when diet is initiated.
Textbook: Page 1472 ANSWER: C

8. The pentalogy of Cantrell includes all of the following except:

A. Epigastric omphalocele.
B. Sternal cleft.
C. Intracardiac defect.
D. Pericardial cyst.
E. Ectopia cordis.

DISCUSSION: The pentalogy of Cantrell includes an epigastric-located omphalocele, ectopia cordis, anterior pleuropericardial defect in the diaphragm, sternal cleft intracardiac defect (most commonly a ventricular septal defect), and, in approximately one third of the cases, a diverticulum of the left ventricle. Pericardial cysts are not part of the pentalogy.
Textbook: Page 1478 ANSWER: D

9. In infants with duodenal atresia, all the following statements are true except:

A. There is an increased incidence of Down's syndrome.
B. It can be detected by prenatal ultrasound examination.
C. It may occur in infants with situs inversus, malrotation, annular pancreas, and anterior portal vein.
D. It is best treated by gastroenterostomy.
E. There is a high incidence of associated cardiac defects.

DISCUSSION: The diagnosis of duodenal atresia can be made prior to the infant's birth with a prenatal ultrasound examination. Infants with duodenal atresia are often premature and have a high incidence of associated anomalies, especially congenital heart disease. Duodenal atresia may also coexist in patients with annular pancreas, situs inversus, malrotation, and anterior portal vein. Approximately one third of the cases occur in babies with Down's syndrome. The operative treatment of choice is a duodenoduodenostomy. Duodenojejunostomy is an alternative procedure. Gastrojejunostomy is not recommended.
Textbook: Page 1469 ANSWER: D

10. The initial treatment of choice for a 2.5-kg infant with a 20-cm-long proximal jejunal atresia and 8 cm of distal ileum is:

A. Laparotomy, nasogastric suction, proximal dilatation to lengthen the atretic jejunum, total parenteral nutrition, and delayed anastomosis.
B. Laparotomy and proximal end-jejunostomy.
C. Laparotomy and immediate small bowel transplantation.
D. Laparotomy and double-barrel enterostomy (jejunum and ileum), with refeeding of jejunal contents into distal ileum and delayed anastomosis.
E. Laparotomy, tapering jejunoplasty, and end-to-oblique jejunoileal anastomosis.

DISCUSSION: The patient has short bowel syndrome with most of the bowel length involving the dilated proximal jejunal atresia. The treatment of choice is to perform a tapering jejunoplasty to preserve bowel length and construct an anastomosis. Early feedings are initiated when bowel function returns in order to stimulate bowel adaptation. Jejunal dilatation does not alter abnormal bowel motility. End-jejunostomy decompresses the obstruction but produces a high ostomy with excessive loss of succus entericus. A double-barrel enterostomy might allow refeeding of jejunal content into the distal ileum and colon, but the proximal atretic loop may have poor function. Small bowel transplantation is not a feasible alternative in the neonate at the present time.
Textbook: Page 1470 ANSWER: E

11. A 2.8-kg neonate with excessive salivation develops respiratory distress. Attempts to pass an orogastric catheter fail because the catheter coils in the back of the throat. A chest film is obtained and shows right upper lobe atelectasis and a gasless abdomen. The most likely diagnosis is:

A. Proximal esophageal atresia without a fistula.
B. Proximal esophageal atresia with a distal tracheoesophageal (TE) fistula.
C. "H-type" TE fistula.
D. Esophageal atresia with both proximal and distal TE fistula.
E. Congenital esophageal stricture.

DISCUSSION: Proximal esophageal atresia results in excess salivation and aspiration of saliva. It is often associated with right upper lobe collapse. Infants with a distal TE fistula have air in the stomach and intestine, as do babies with both proximal and distal fistulas, H-type fistula, and an esophageal stricture. Infants with proximal atresia but without a TE fistula do not have air beneath the diaphragm. Attempts at passing an orogastric catheter are met by an obstruction and coiling of the catheter in the infant's mouth. The catheter passes into the stomach in infants with H-type TE fistula and in most infants with esophageal stricture.
Textbook: Page 1467 ANSWER: A

12. Neonates with necrotizing enterocolitis (NEC) may demonstrate all of the following findings on abdominal films except:

A. Pneumatosis intestinalis.
B. Portal vein air.
C. Pneumoperitoneum.

D. Colovesical fistula.
E. Fixed and thickened bowel loops.

DISCUSSION: Infants with NEC do not develop a colovesical fistula as an initial x-ray finding. Pneumatosis, portal vein air, pneumoperitoneum, and fixed intestinal loops with thickened bowel wall are all observed with some regularity in babies with NEC.
Textbook: Page 1476 ANSWER: D

13. The most common type of congenital diaphragmatic hernia is caused by:

A. A defect in the central tendon.
B. Eventration of the diaphragm in the fetus.
C. A defect through the space of Larrey.
D. An abnormally wide esophageal hiatus.
E. A defect through the pleuroperitoneal fold.

DISCUSSION: Eventration of the diaphragm is related to phrenic nerve paralysis. It is more commonly observed after a breech delivery and may be associated with torticollis and Erb's palsy. The space of Larrey is located anteriorly just off the midline. A Morgagni hernia passes through this potential space. An abnormally wide esophageal hiatus would most likely create a sliding hiatal hernia. The most common type of congenital diaphragmatic hernia in the neonate is the posterolateral Bochdalek hernia, which passes through a defect in the developing pleuroperitoneal fold.
Textbook: Page 1480 ANSWER: E

14. The calorie-nitrogen ratio for an infant should be maintained at:

A. 75:1.
B. 100:1.
C. 50:1.
D. 150:1.
E. 25:1.

DISCUSSION: The calorie-nitrogen ratio should be maintained at 150:1 for most infants. Fever, major illness, sepsis, or trauma may increase the caloric requirements significantly.
Textbook: Page 1466 ANSWER: D

15. All of the following conditions are derived from the primitive embryologic foregut except:

A. Bronchogenic cyst.
B. Cystic adenomatoid malformation.
C. Gastric duplication.
D. Mesenteric cyst.
E. Pulmonary sequestration.

DISCUSSION: Mesenteric cysts are derived from lymphatic anlage in the abdomen and are unassociated with foregut development. The lung buds arise from the primitive foregut, and anomalies associated with tracheopulmonary development are therefore all derived from the foregut. These include tracheoesophageal fistula, congenital lobar emphysema, enteric cysts (which may communicate with the normal esophagus, lung, or spinal canal; e.g., neurenteric cyst), cystic adenomatoid malformations, solitary lung cysts, intra- and extralobar sequestrations, and bronchogenic cysts. The stomach and first part of the duodenum are also of foregut origin, and thus a gastric duplication is by definition derived from the foregut.
Textbook: Page 1488 ANSWER: D

NOTES

NOTES

CHAPTER 17

NEUROSURGERY

1. Lumbar disc disease is a common cause of pain in adults. Which of the following statements regarding this condition is true?

A. Weakness of the anterior longitudinal ligament over the lateral aspect of the intervertebral disc results in a susceptibility to tearing with resulting disc herniation and compression of a nerve root or the cauda equina.
B. Central herniation of the L3–L4 disc typically results in spinal cord compression and bilateral lower extremity weakness.
C. A left L5–S1 disc herniation usually compresses the left S1 nerve root.
D. Neurogenic claudication can be distinguished from vascular claudication because of the fact that symptoms in neurogenic claudication frequently improve with the resumption of activity.

DISCUSSION: Clinically, herniated discs at one level usually affect the disc that exits at the next level below. In normal circumstances, a herniated disc at the L5–S1 level compresses the S1 nerve root as it exits the dural sac. In a similar fashion, a disc herniation at the L4–L5 level typically results in an L5 radiculopathy. Although disc herniations can occur in any direction, those that occur posterolaterally are more likely to be clinically significant due to the proximity of the nerve roots that are exiting through the neural foramina and the cauda equina within the dural sac. Large, central disc herniations are known to result in bilateral symptoms. Since the caudal extent of the spinal cord in most individuals is found at the L1–L2 disc space, compression of the cauda equina and not the spinal cord is more likely to occur in an L3–L4 disc herniation. The pain associated with neurogenic claudication is characteristically relieved soon after the patient sits down. Standing and walking tend to evoke symptoms, whereas flexion of the spine or leaning forward tends to relieve them.

Textbook: Page 1534 ANSWER: C

2. Neural tube defects occur in various forms and result from disordered embryogenesis. Which of the following statements regarding neural tube defects is true?

A. Myelomeningoceles occur as a result of disordered retrogressive differentiation and are typically associated with malformed genitalia, imperforate anus, and renal dysplasias.
B. Children with lipomyelomeningocele typically present with a skin-covered midline soft tissue mass.
C. Myelomeningoceles can occur in any region of the spine but the more rostral portions are the most commonly affected.
D. The majority of children with lipomyelomeningoceles develop hydrocephalus.

DISCUSSION: Lipomyelomeningoceles occur due to a disorder of caudal neural tube formation. These disorders are frequently referred to as occult dysraphic states because they form beneath intact dermal elements. Patients with lipomyelomeningoceles typically present with a midline soft tissue mass and occasionally with cutaneous dimples or hemangiomas. Disorders of caudal neural tube formation may also occur as part of a broader *caudal regression syndrome,* which may be associated with imperforate anus, malformed genitalia, or renal dysplasias. Myelomeningoceles result from a defect in the process of primary neurulation. This failure of neural tube closure results in an incomplete meningeal and dermal covering of the spinal cord and the presence of an exposed neural placode in surviving children. Although myelomeningoceles may affect any region of the spine, the thoracolumbar and lumbar segments predominate. Nearly every child born with a myelomeningocele also has a Chiari II malformation. Between 80 and 90% of these children develop hydrocephalus and require ventriculoperitoneal shunting.

Textbook: Page 1544 ANSWER: B

3. All of the following primary brain tumors commonly infiltrate into surrounding brain except:

A. Glioblastoma.
B. Oligodendroglioma.
C. Meningioma.
D. Low-grade astrocytoma.
E. Ependymoma.

DISCUSSION: All primary tumors derived from glial cells infiltrate into surrounding brain tissue. Glioblastomas and low-grade astrocytomas derive from astrocytes, oligodendrogliomas derive from oligodendrocytes, and ependymomas derive from ependymal cells. This characteristic to infiltrate makes a surgical cure for gliomas impossible because tumor cells are inevitably left behind in the relatively normal brain surrounding the tumor resection cavity. Meningiomas are benign, extra-axial (outside the brain) tumors derived from arachnoidal cap cells that may be cured with complete resection. Only in the rare situation of a malignant meningioma does this tumor infiltrate into the brain.

Textbook: Page 1525 ANSWER: C

4. A patient with a nonfunctional, pituitary macroadenoma that is elevating the optic chiasm and causing diminished vision is best treated by:

A. Transsphenoidal craniotomy.
B. Gamma knife radiosurgery.
C. Dopamine agonist therapy.
D. Fractionated radiation therapy.
E. Methotrexate.

DISCUSSION: The best treatment for a pituitary macroadenoma that is causing visual symptoms is surgical resection. The most effective approach to the pituitary gland is via a transsphenoidal craniotomy. No brain retraction is necessary and morbidity is minimized. Radiosurgery is less effective against large pituitary tumors because the proximity of the optic chiasm hinders the amount of radiation that can be delivered. Only functional adenomas secreting prolactin are responsive to dopamine agonist therapy. Fractionated radiation therapy is unlikely to reduce mass effect and will not improve visual symptoms. The potential toxicity of chemotherapy such as methotrexate contraindicates its usage.

Textbook: Page 1527 ANSWER: A

5. C6 radiculopathy is clinically characterized by which of the following?

A. Motor weakness (flexion of the elbow).
B. Diminished biceps reflex.
C. Numbness in thumb and index finger.
D. All of the above.

DISCUSSION: The C6 nerve root is the most common nerve root affected in cervical radiculopathy and is characterized by radicular arm pain, pain at the scapula tip, numbness in the thumb and index finger, weakness flexion of the elbow, and weakness in extension of the wrist.

Textbook: Page 1536 ANSWER: D

6. If subarachnoid hemorrhage is suspected in a drowsy patient, which of the following would be the procedure of choice to confirm the diagnosis?

A. Magnetic resonance imaging (MRI) of the brain.
B. Computed tomography (CT) of the brain.
C. Angiogram.
D. Lumbar puncture.

DISCUSSION: In a drowsy patient with a suspected subarachnoid hemorrhage, space-occupying hematomas might be present, and therefore a CT scan is indicated prior to performing a lumbar puncture to prevent herniation. MRI is not as accurate as a CT scan to detect early subarachnoid hemorrhage. An angiogram is only performed following confirmation of a subarachnoid hemorrhage to establish the cause.

Textbook: Page 1519 ANSWER: B

NOTES

NOTES

CHAPTER 18

PLASTIC SURGERY

1. The most important dimension of wound contraction in terms of appearance and function is:

A. Longitudinal (same axis as wound).
B. Transverse (axis is perpendicular to wound).
C. Plane is perpendicular to surface of wound.
D. A wound contracts equally in all dimensions.

DISCUSSION: A wound contracts up to 20% in the longitudinal axis. This is the most important reason that scars become functionally limiting or unsightly. Because the transverse dimension is such a short distance, it does not usually contribute significantly to aesthetic appearance or functional impairment. Contraction in the dimension perpendicular to the surface of the wound does not contribute to functional impairment, but it can cause depression of the scar. Using everting sutures or eversion by design of the excision prevents scar depression.
Textbook: Pages 1550–1551 ANSWER: A

2. The skin layer that contributes the most to breaking strength in a linear closure is:

A. Epidermis.
B. Dermis.
C. Subcutaneous fat.
D. Each layer contributes equally.

DISCUSSION: The organized collagen structure of the dermis provides most of the strength in wound closure. Epidermal sutures are used only for fine approximation of the skin edges. Subcutaneous fat does not hold sutures well. Moreover sutures placed in the subcutaneous fat can serve as a nidus for infection.
Textbook: Pages 1551–1552 ANSWER: B

3. Which absorbable suture retains its tensile strength longest?

A. Plain catgut.
B. Chromic gut.
C. Polyglecaprone.
D. They retain their strength equally.

DISCUSSION: Plain catgut is a twisted filament that loses most of its tensile strength in 7 to 10 days. Chromic gut, which is gut that has been tanned in chromic acid, retains its tensile strength for about twice as long. Polyglecaprone is a monofilament that retains its tensile strength for 3 to 4 weeks. It provokes a much smaller tissue reaction than does gut and it is very pliable and easy to use. In general, fast-absorbing sutures are used for approximation of mucosa, while slow-absorbing sutures are preferred for approximation of the dermis.
Textbook: Pages 1552–1553 ANSWER: C

4. How much time does it take a wound to achieve 100% of its tissue tensile strength?

A. 1 week.
B. 1 month.
C. 1 year.
D. Never.

DISCUSSION: Although the strength of a wound gets stronger with time as collagen absorption and deposition leads to greater organization, the tissue never achieves 100% of its prewounding tensile strength. Years later, it will have regained only 80 to 90% of its original strength.
Textbook: Page 1552 ANSWER: D

5. How should a contaminated wound be irrigated?

A. Gently running saline over it so as not to further damage tissue.
B. Running saline around the perimeter of the wound while avoiding the deepest parts of the wound so as not to spread contamination to deeper tissue.
C. Pulsatile jet lavage to all layers of the wound.
D. Using a saline-soaked gauze to wash only the areas of the wound that are visibly contaminated.

DISCUSSION: Every wound that is not electively created in a sterile environment should be considered contaminated and should be irrigated with copious amounts of saline using pulsatile jet lavage. Care should be taken to irrigate all parts of the wound including the deepest tissue laayers.
Textbook: Pages 1550–1553 ANSWER: C

6. Which type of skin graft results in the greatest amount of wound contraction?

A. Partial-thickness skin graft.
B. Ful-thickness skin graft.
C. No skin graft.
D. They all contract equally.

DISCUSSION: The thicker the skin graft, the less wound contraction. Thus, a wound treated with a full-thickness skin graft contracts less than one treated with a partial-thickness skin graft. A wound that receives no graft, but is left to heal by contraction and re-epithelialization, will have the greatest amount of wound contraction.

Textbook: Pages 1553–1554 ANSWER: C

7. The process whereby capillaries from a skin graft become aligned with capillaries from the recipient bed is called:

A. Inosculation.
B. Imbibition.
C. Reanastomosis.
D. Revascularization.

DISCUSSION: *Imbibition* refers to absorption of nutrients into the graft through the recipient bed capillaries, which serves to feed the graft for the first 24 to 48 hours. *Inosculation* is the process whereby donor and recipient capillaries become aligned. During the first two phases, the graft becomes adhered to the recipient bed by fibrous deposition at the interface. In the third phase, *revascularization* is completed by differentiation of the connecting vessels into arterioles and venules. It is not known whether growth of new vessels into the graft or the growing together of donor and host vessels is the primary mechanism for *revascularization.*

Textbook: Page 1553 ANSWER: A

8. What is the most common cause of graft failure?

A. Infection.
B. Motions.
C. Blood clot.
D. Fluid between the graft and recipient bed.

DISCUSSION: If the graft becomes separated from the recipient bed by fluid (hematoma or seroma), it will not take. This is the most common cause of graft failure. One way of avoiding the collection of fluid under a graft is to mesh it. By creating multiple incisions in the graft, drainage is allowed. Meshing also allows the graft to become expandable, so it can be used to cover a larger defect. However, a meshed graft creates a "pebbled" appearance when it has healed and is not as aesthetically acceptable, particularly in the face and the hand.

Textbook: Page 1554 ANSWER: D

9. What is the most common cause of facial paralysis?

A. Bell's palsy.
B. Neoplasm.
C. Trauma.
D. Multiple sclerosis.

DISCUSSION: The most common diagnosis in patients with facial paralysis is Bell's palsy. The incidence of Bell's palsy in the United States is 20 per 100,000 population per year. It is commonly associated with pregnancy and diabetes mellitus.

Textbook: Page 1558 ANSWER: A

10. What percentage of lower extremity ulcers can be healed with a conservative wound care program consisting of débridement, optimal dressings, and compression?

A. 30%.
B. 50%.
C. 70%.
D. 90%.

DISCUSSION: For about half of lower extremity ulcers, healing can be achieved through nonoperative management. Healing is promoted by the removal of devitalized and contaminated tissue, hydrated dressings to prevent desiccation, and compression. If the ulcer is over a bony prominence, it increases the likelihood that surgery will be necessary.

Textbook: Page 1565 ANSWER: B

11. Most cleft lip protocols call for repair at what age?

A. 3 months.
B. 1 year.
C. 3 years.
D. 6 years.

DISCUSSION: Most treatment protocols call for repair of the cleft lip at approximately 3 months, the cleft palate at approximately 6 months, and for bone grafting of the deficient alveolar bone at approximately 9 years. Many surgeons prefer to do a lip adhesion 1 to 2 months before the definitive lip repair in order to optimize the quality of the repair. The repair of the soft palate facilitates the development of normal speech, but the repair of the hard palate negatively influences midfacial growth. Some treatment protocols, therefore, call for early repair of the soft palate and late repair of the hard palate. If necessary, an obturator is used in the hard palate until it is repaired, in order to facilitate speech.

Textbook: Page 1557 ANSWER: A

12. If possible, elective incisions should be avoided in what anatomic area?

A. Submandibular area.
B. Plantar surface of feet.
C. Flank area.
D. Retroauricular area.

DISCUSSION: Incisions in the plantar area of the foot should be avoided because temporary or permanent pain with scarring is a common problem. Incisions on the shoulders or in the triangle over the anterior chest that is created by the acromion processes and the xiphoid process should also be avoided, because incisions in these areas often heal with a hypertrophic or keloidal scar.

Textbook: Page 1550 ANSWER: B

13. Sutures in the eyelid should be removed after how many days?

A. 3 to 4 days.
B. 7 to 8 days.

C. 11 to 12 days.
D. 2 weeks.

DISCUSSION: The longer a transepidermal suture is left in, the greater the scarring. Sutures in the face are left in for a relatively shorter length of time because the face is not subjected to the same stretching and shearing forces as other parts of the body and because the aesthetic appearance of a scar is of greater importance in the face.

Textbook: Pages 1552–1553 ANSWER: A

NOTES

NOTES

NOTES

CHAPTER 19

ORTHOPAEDICS

1. What is the most common tumor of the hand?

A. Ganglion.
B. Giant cell tumor.
C. Epidermal inclusion cyst.
D. Lipoma.

DISCUSSION: Ganglion cyst is the most common soft tissue tumor in the hand. The others listed are some of the remaining more common types found in the hand.

Textbook: Page 1581 ANSWER: A

2. The most common carpal bone fracture is:

A. Scaphoid.
B. Capitate.
C. Lunate.
D. Hamate.

DISCUSSION: The scaphoid bone fracture may not be visualized by x-ray until several weeks after injury. Therefore, a high index of suspicion on clinical examination warrants splint immobilization of the wrist for 6 to 8 weeks for healing.

Textbook: Pages 1576–1577 ANSWER: A

3. The most common congenital hand anomaly is:

A. Duplication.
B. Brachydactyly.
C. Polydactyly.
D. Syndactyly.

DISCUSSION: Syndactyly is most prevalent in the Western hemisphere; polydactyly is most prevalent in Africa.

Textbook: Pages 1583–1584 ANSWER: D

4. Where is the most common anatomic site of trigger finger?

A. Annular pulley V.
B. Annular pulley IV.
C. Annular pulley II.
D. Annular pulley III.
E. Annular pulley I.

DISCUSSION: Triggering usually occurs at the first annular pulley. It can be relieved by splinting and steroid injections and may require surgical release of the annular I pulley in order to relieve the triggering.

Textbook: Page 1585 ANSWER: E

5. Name the dorsal compartment of the wrist that contains the extensor tendon to the thumb.

A. Compartment I.
B. Compartment II.
C. Compartment III.
D. Compartment IV.
E. Compartment V.
F. Compartment VI.

DISCUSSION: The extensor compartments located on the dorsal side of the wrist are important for the clinical mechanics of the tendon mechanisms. Lacerations and injuries to these areas require knowledge of the compartments and the occupying structures in order to restore proper function to the hand following injury.

Compartment I	Extensor pollicis brevis tendon Abductor pollicis longus tendon
Compartment II	Extensor carpi radialis longus tendon Extensor carpi radialis brevis tendon
Compartment III	Extensor pollicis longus tendon
Compartment IV	Extensor indicis proprius tendon Extensor digitorum communis tendon
Compartment V	Extensor digiti quinti tendon
Compartment VI	Extensor carpi ulnaris tendon

Textbook: Pages 1572–1575 ANSWER: C

6. A 22-year-old woman who was a front-seat passenger in a head-on motor vehicle accident sustained an anterior-posterior compression-type pelvic ring injury with 7 cm of pubic symphysis widening. She is hemodynamically unstable after adequate fluid resuscitation. The trauma room chest radiograph and the diagnostic peritoneal lavage are negative. The next step in her management is:

A. External fixation of the unstable pelvic ring injury.
B. Laparotomy with pelvic packing.
C. Angiography with potential embolization of the pelvic vessels.
D. Open reduction and internal fixation of the pelvic injury.
E. Continued blood and fluid support and expectant observation.

DISCUSSION: Anterior-posterior compression-type injuries with more than 2.5 cm of diastasis are considered unstable. Once all sources of bleeding are ruled out, external fixation—either with a pelvic clamp or a resuscitation-type external fixator frame—is the next step in controlling hemorrhage and stabilizing the patient. Arterial bleeding is present in only 10% of the cases, and angiography is successful in a fraction of these cases.

Textbook: Pages 1598–1602 ANSWER: A

7. Three hours after sustaining a closed tibial shaft fracture in a fall from a roof, a 35-year-old man has excruciating pain in his anterolateral leg despite narcotic analgesics. His compartments are tense and palpation causes exquisite pain. Passive flexion of his toes causes severe pain in his leg and calf. Sensation is intact in his foot and his pulses are strong. Given this examination, the patient should now undergo:

A. Continued observation and an increase in his narcotics.
B. Removal of his posterior splint and recasting of the extremity.
C. Emergent four-compartment fasciotomy using a two-incision technique.
D. Repeat radiographs to rule out an additional occult fracture.
E. Compartment pressure measurement using a hand-held manometer.

DISCUSSION: Fasciotomies are indicated when the clinical examination clearly demonstrates the findings of a developing compartment syndrome. Compartment pressure measurements are not necessary in cases in which the clinical findings are unequivocal.

Textbook: Pages 1604–1609 ANSWER: C

8. All of the following patient outcomes are improved with immediate stabilization (within 24 hours) of femoral shaft fractures in the multiply injured patient except the:

A. Development of the adult respiratory distress syndrome (ARDS).
B. Rate of venous thromboembolic events.
C. Need for narcotic analgesia.
D. Time to union of the fracture.
E. Formation of decubitus ulcers.

DISCUSSION: Outcomes related to the healing of the fracture are unaffected by immediate versus delayed stabilization. ARDS, deep venous thrombosis, decubitus ulcers, and the need for narcotics are decreased when femoral shaft fractures are stabilized immediately.

Textbook: Pages 1613–1614 ANSWER: D

9. A 58-year-old man sustained a Type IIIA open tibial fracture in a motorcycle accident. There is gross contamination of the wound with gravel. After the patient is stabilized:

A. Broad-spectrum antibiotics are given, and a sterile dressing and a splint are applied with the decision regarding final stabilization to be made by the attending orthopaedic staff in the morning.
B. No antibiotics are given until after cultures are obtained in the operating room prior to emergent irrigation and aggressive débridement.
C. Irrigation should be carried out in the emergency room and a cast applied.
D. Broad-spectrum antibiotics and tetanus prophylaxis are administered, and emergent irrigation and débridement in the operating room are performed.
E. The wound should be cleaned of all debris and wet-to-dry dressings applied every shift.

DISCUSSION: Emergency room management of open fractures consists of administration of broad-spectrum antibiotics, tetanus prophylaxis, and sterile dressing of the wound. If there is soil contamination, penicillin can be added to cover clostridial species. Emergent irrigation and débridement are mandatory in this contaminated fracture if the patient's overall condition allows.

Textbook: Pages 1609–1612 ANSWER: D

10. A 48-year-old woman sustained a posterior knee dislocation in a motor vehicle accident. There are weak distal pulses palpable in the affected leg. After reduction, the pulse returns and is strong. Which of the following best describes the most appropriate management of this patient?

A. The knee is immobilized, and no further management is necessary.
B. The knee is immobilized, and the ligamentous injury is addressed urgently.
C. The knee is immobilized, and the patient should be taken to the operating room for repair of the vascular occlusion.
D. The knee is immobilized, and angiography is performed with the early involvement of the vascular surgery team.
E. No immobilization is necessary.

DISCUSSION: Posterior knee dislocations are commonly associated with popliteal artery injuries. An intimal flap tear may be present and distal pulses still palpable. Angiography is considered mandatory in all posterior knee dislocations. On-table angiography is generally considered unreliable and is unnecessary in a patient with palpable pulses and a currently viable foot.

Textbook: Pages 1602–1604 ANSWER: D

NOTES

NOTES

CHAPTER 20

GYNECOLOGY

1. All of the following statements about the ureter in the female pelvis are true except:

A. It enters the pelvis at the level of the common iliac artery.
B. It passes downward on the lateral pelvic side wall.
C. It passes about 1.5 cm lateral to the exterior of the cervix.
D. It passes over the uterine artery.
E. It derives its blood supply from the renal, ovarian, hypogastric, and inferior vesical arteries.

DISCUSSION: The figure in the textbook displays the relationship of the uterine artery to the ureter. It is important to know that the uterine artery passes over the ureter so that one may more effectively avoid it during hysterectomy. The important issue is to clamp close to the uterus and so avoid this important structure.

Textbook: Page 1623 ANSWER: D

2. All of the following statements about the blood supply to the female pelvic reproductive structures (uterus, vagina, fallopian tubes, ovaries) are correct except:

A. The ovarian arteries arise from the aorta, just below the renal arteries.
B. The right ovarian vein empties into the vena cava, and the left ovarian vein drains into the left renal vein.
C. The internal iliac vessels are 3 to 4 cm in length.
D. The internal pudendal artery is the most caudal extension of the hypogastric artery.
E. The vulvar erectile tissues are supplied by the vaginal artery.

DISCUSSION: The internal arterial support to the pelvic structures is important. It appears that the vulvar-rectal tissues are primarily supported by the vaginal branch of the uterine artery.

Textbook: Page 1623 ANSWER: E

3. All of the following statements about the female neuroendocrine system are correct except:

A. The ovary only becomes responsive to follicle-stimulating hormone (FSH) and luteinizing hormone (LH) at puberty.
B. The hypothalamus serves as the primary control system.
C. Gonadotropin-releasing hormone must be produced in a pulsatile fashion to properly cause gonadotropin synthesis and release.
D. Estrogen, progesterone, and inhibin modulate pituitary gonadotropin release.
E. Neurotransmitters control hypothalamic function.

DISCUSSION: The ovary is responsive to FSH and LH at any age, including prior to puberty. The hypothalamus serves as the primary control system, and its maturation is important in the pubertal process. Once estrogen is present, pubertal changes begin to occur.

Textbook: Pages 1624–1626 ANSWER: A

4. The following statements are true about carcinoma of the cervix except:

A. Premalignant lesions cannot be detected by Pap smear.
B. Ninety-five percent of cervical carcinomas are squamous cancers.
C. Therapy is based on histology and staging.
D. Therapeutic options include surgery and irradiation.
E. Cervical carcinoma can cause ureteral obstruction.

DISCUSSION: Cervical cancer is the second most common gynecologic malignancy. Premalignant lesions can be detected by Pap smears, but not always. There is an intrinsic failure rate in the Pap smear that approaches 30%. The remainder of the answers are correct as they relate to cervical cancer.

Textbook: Pages 1633–1637 ANSWER: A

5. The following statements are true about ovarian cancer except:

A. It accounts for approximately 5% of all malignancies in women.
B. The majority are germ cell tumors.
C. In only 20% of patients does earlier detection allow for complete surgical removal.
D. Pap smears are useful in detection.
E. It may be associated with recurrent small bowel obstruction.

DISCUSSION: The majority of malignancies of the ovary are epidermoid lesions, although a small minority are due to germ cell tumors. Pap smears are invariably useful in detection, and ovarian cancer is often associated with small bowel obstruction.

Textbook: Pages 1641–1642 ANSWER: B

6. The following statements about patients with ectopic pregnancy are true except:

A. The incidence is increasing.
B. The likelihood of a pregnancy being ectopic is increased in patients with prior pelvic surgery, conception with in vitro fertilization (IVF), and pregnancy after tubal sterilization.
C. These patients rarely have a positive pregnancy test.
D. Ectopic pregnancy can usually be visualized by transvaginal ultrasound when human chorionic gonadotropin (hCG) is 2000 mIU/ml or less.

DISCUSSION: Ectopic gestation is increasing in incidence. The likelihood of an ectopic pregnancy is associated with prior pelvic surgery, conception by IVF, pregnancy after tubal sterilization, and other causes. A woman with an ectopic pregnancy usually has a positive pregnancy test, and when the hCG is 2000 mIU/ml or less, one can often see the ectopic pregnancy by ultrasound. Of major importance, however, is that when the hCG is about 2000 mIU/ml, one should surely be able to see an intrauterine pregnancy. Thus, an "empty" uterus on ultrasound when hCG is 2000 mIU/ml or more is highly associated with ectopic pregnancy.

Textbook: Pages 1643–1644 ANSWER: C

7. Physiologic changes in pregnant women include all of the following except:

A. Decreased gastric and intestinal motility.
B. Increased plasma volume with a lesser increase of red blood cells (RBCs).
C. Decreased cardiac work.
D. Thyroid gland hyperplasia.
E. Doubling in size of the pituitary.

DISCUSSION: Physiologic changes in pregnant women include decreased gastric and intestinal motility and increased plasma volume. There is an associated, lesser increase of RBCs. Thyroid gland hyperplasia occurs primarily due to the stimulation of human chorionic thyrotropin. The pituitary usually increases in size during pregnancy. Increased cardiac work is noted as a pregnancy change.

Textbook: Pages 1644–1645 ANSWER: C

NOTES

NOTES

CHAPTER 21

UROLOGY

1. The site of conversion of calcidiol to calcitriol is the:

A. Proximal tubule.
B. Distal tubule.
C. Juxtaglomerular apparatus.
D. Collecting duct.

DISCUSSION: The proximal tubule is the site of conversion of calcidiol to calcitriol. Calcitriol is one of the most potent stimulators of intestinal calcium absorption and a metabolite of vitamin D_3.

Textbook: Pages 1653–1654 ANSWER: A

2. Which is not a normal anatomic site of narrowing along the course of the ureter?

A. The ureteropelvic junction.
B. The crossing of the iliac vessels.
C. The ureterovesical junction.
D. The entrance to the true pelvis.

DISCUSSION: From proximal to distal, the normal anatomic sites of narrowing are the ureteropelvic junction, the crossing of the iliac vessels, and the ureterovesical junction. These are common locations for hang-up of a ureteral calculus during passage.

Textbook: Pages 1649–1652 ANSWER: D

3. Which is not a urologic manifestation of von Hippel–Lindau disease?

A. Renal tumors.
B. Renal cysts.
C. Transitional cell carcinoma.
D. Epididymal cystadenomas.

DISCUSSION: Von Hippel–Lindau disease is associated with renal tumors and cysts, pheochromocytomas, and epididymal cystadenomas. Other nonurologic manifestations include cerebellar and spinal hemangioblastomas, retinal hemangiomas, and pancreatic islet cell tumors.

Textbook: Page 1660 ANSWER: C

NOTES

NOTES

NOTES